WELL-CHILD CARE IN INFANCY

WELL-CHILD CARE IN INFANCY

Promoting Readiness for Life

William B. Pittard III, MD, PhD, MPH

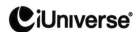

WELL-CHILD CARE IN INFANCY
PROMOTING READINESS FOR LIFE

Copyright © 2016 William Pittard.

All rights reserved. No part of this book may be used or reproduced by any means, graphic, electronic, or mechanical, including photocopying, recording, taping or by any information storage retrieval system without the written permission of the author except in the case of brief quotations embodied in critical articles and reviews.

iUniverse books may be ordered through booksellers or by contacting:

iUniverse
1663 Liberty Drive
Bloomington, IN 47403
www.iuniverse.com
1-800-Authors (1-800-288-4677)

Because of the dynamic nature of the Internet, any web addresses or links contained in this book may have changed since publication and may no longer be valid. The views expressed in this work are solely those of the author and do not necessarily reflect the views of the publisher, and the publisher hereby disclaims any responsibility for them.

Any people depicted in stock imagery provided by Thinkstock are models, and such images are being used for illustrative purposes only. Certain stock imagery © Thinkstock.

ISBN: 978-1-4917-8228-6 (sc)
ISBN: 978-1-4917-8227-9 (e)

Library of Congress Control Number: 2015919138

Print information available on the last page.

iUniverse rev. date: 01/28/2016

To my wife, Judith Dowty Pittard, who has supported my academic efforts for more than forty-three years; to James N. and Sarah B. Laditka, who served on my PhD dissertation committee and provided both pre- and postdoctoral public-health guidance and understanding necessary for this book; and to John H. Kennell and Marshal H. Klaus, who individually served as surrogate fathers to me throughout my neonatal-perinatal training and early academic career.

Contents

Foreword ix
Preface xi
Chapter 1 Well-Child Care: Components, Benefits, History, and Future Need 1
Chapter 2 Continuity of Care 13
Chapter 3 Well-Child Care Screening 23
Chapter 4 Well-Child Care Parental Anticipatory Guidance in the Preschool Years: Clinical Effectiveness 52
Chapter 5 Routine Immunizations Birth to Six Years: Clinical Effectiveness 67
Chapter 6 Well-Child Care in a Changing US Delivery System 85
Chapter 7 Well-Child Care: A Prudent Investment for the Future 98
About the Authors 117
About the Book 121
Notes 123
Index 163

Foreword

Over 150 years ago, author Charles Dickens made note that close to half of the coffins being made in England in the mid-1800s were sized for children. Today, relatively few children in the United States die from disease or accidents. Pediatricians are the true champions of disease and accident prevention. They have worked persistently to research and improve nutrition, disease prevention, medications, vaccines, accident prevention, parental guidance and education, and the importance of a nurturing environment. Without question, these preventative measures are why children today are healthy and why, thankfully, there is little need for small coffins in our country.

The authors of this book have compiled a comprehensive synopsis of best practices in preventive pediatric medicine. This volume sets forth the recognized standards of care for children. Although children in the United States generally have access to health care meeting these standards, it is an unfortunate fact that many children living elsewhere do not. As a profession, we should take on the endeavor of providing standards-based care to all children across the world—and reduce the need for small coffins everywhere.

Children's hospitals and their specialized staff may dramatically save a child's life on occasion. But keep in mind that primary care physicians, practicing preventive medicine on a daily basis, have the greatest impact on children's health. It is these physicians who are responsible for saving thousands of lives each and every year.

Charles P. Darby Jr., MD
Professor Emeritus of Pediatrics
Medical University of South Carolina
Charleston, South Carolina
September 18, 2013

Preface

Well-child care represents preventive health services for children provided by physicians and other health-care providers. These services include screening for normal growth and visual, hearing, and social/emotional development, immunizations, and parental child-health education and reassurance, often referred to as parental anticipatory guidance. Although preventive care for children serves as a health-care paradigm today and is broadly accepted by providers and parents as something of paramount importance for normal child development, utilization has been limited for more affluent children by high co-pay insurance requirements and for low-income children, where care is government funded, by lack of awareness of its availability and the benefit to children.

Empiric documentation of clinical effectiveness for well-child care, other than for immunizations, has been extremely slow in development. As far back as 1973, the American Academy of Pediatrics (AAP) recognized this information gap and requested that investigators address this issue. Nevertheless, effectiveness for the nonimmunization well-child care components has been reported only in the last six years. The difficulty created by this lack of information was compounded by an Institute of Medicine (IOM) report in 1990 indicating that correcting the underuse of needed health care, such as well-child services, while increasing the quality of care, tends to be associated with increased cost. Therefore, although public- and private-insurance administrators want improved quality of care, with clinical effectiveness unproven and cost likely to be increased, their incentive to implement methods to increase well-child care utilization has been limited.

This book on well-child care has been written for individual and population health-care workers interested in the well-being of children. Thus, the primary stakeholders include parents, health-care providers, and health-insurance/Medicaid policy makers

William B. Pittard III, MD, PhD, MPH

and administrators. The purpose of this book is to increase awareness in all stakeholders but particularly in health-insurance administrators of the preventive-care benefits for preschool children to facilitate the implementation of methods to increase well-child care utilization and improve health status for children.

Although well-child care immunization data are included in this book, the focus is on the more recent findings confirming clinical effectiveness for the nonimmunization or screening, developmental assessment, and parental anticipatory guidance components.

Each chapter author is an accomplished child-care specialist with several years of clinical experience. The book serves to close the information gap created by the long delay in confirming clinical effectiveness for well-child care. By summarizing the more recent findings, this book provides justification for the potential added costs to well-child care provision by introducing methods to increase preventive-care utilization. Each chapter is written to be read in a stand-alone fashion, with some recognized background information redundancy between chapters. The book first provides an overview of well-child care history and benefits and explores the specific elements of well-child care (continuity/quality, screening, parental anticipatory guidance, and immunizations). Then it addresses the influence of government policies and private-sector primary care provider (PCP) health-care delivery, offering ideas for improved care. Last, chapter 7 summarizes and discusses how available outcome data indicate preschool well-child care is a prudent investment for the future of children.

CHAPTER 1

Well-Child Care: Components, Benefits, History, and Future Need

William B. Pittard III, MD, PhD, MPH

Introduction

Well-child care is designed to promote optimal physical, social, and cognitive development for children from birth through twenty years. A broadly accepted manifestation of success for this preventive care in the preschool years is increased time without illness and readiness for first-grade learning. Increased wellness time should promote greater opportunity for playing and interacting with other children and adults, facilitating socialization, school readiness, and more long-term life success.[1] Specifically, well-child visits in the preschool years include an assessment of physical growth, anticipatory guidance for parents or caregivers, immunizations, and screening procedures for illness and abnormal vision, hearing, and cognitive development.[2]

The book first provides an overview of well-child care, describing its components and anticipated benefits for children. The history of governmental recognition of need for well-child care and its funding for low-income children includes the Children's Bureau; the Sheppard-Towner Act; the American Academy of Pediatrics (AAP); Medicaid and the confrontations and controversies surrounding its early and periodic screening, diagnosis, and treatment (EPSDT) benefit for children; and the establishment of the State Children's Health Insurance Program (SCHIP). The chapter concludes with a look at future needs for maternal and child preventive care.

William B. Pittard III, MD, PhD, MPH

Components and Benefits

Well-child visits offer clinicians an opportunity to identify and address problems that might impede optimal growth and development. The AAP recommends frequent well-child/EPSDT visits in the preschool years, including six visits in year one, three visits in year two, two in year three, and one visit annually thereafter.[3] An initial visit during the prenatal period provides child-health education and anticipatory guidance for soon-to-be parents, and postdelivery visits offer age-appropriate immunizations, developmental and sensory evaluations, assessment of nutrition status and oral health, and age-specific parenting education. Parents of children with the recommended number of visits in infancy should receive more information than parents of children with fewer visits about cognitive stimulation for their children and about avoiding risks to cognitive health, such as lead exposure, accidents, and undernutrition.[4] Recommended topics for parental anticipatory guidance include advice regarding physical activity, appropriate use of health-care services, parent-child reading, and avoidance of household toxins.[5] Developmental screening includes assessment of height and weight, vision, hearing, language skills, and behavior; the screening is designed to facilitate the early implementation of corrective measures for any abnormality detected with improved health outcomes.[6]

Despite the benefits of well-child care, it is not always utilized. Due to cost and lack of information confirming well-child care effectiveness, privately insured children have been reported to underuse well-child care, particularly in the preschool years.[7] In contrast, despite government funding, the Medicaid EPSDT/well-child benefit is more likely to be underutilized by low-income children than well-child care by privately insured children.[8]

Although providing well-child care involves cost, not using well-child visits often results in still greater medical costs. Low-income children also more frequently use emergency department and in-hospital, nonprimary care provider services for nonurgent ambulatory care sensitive condition (ACSC) diagnoses than higher income children.[9] ACSC diagnoses include asthma; seizure; cellulitis; ear, nose, and throat infections; bacterial pneumonia;

kidney and urinary tract infections; and gastrointestinal infections and are illnesses routinely treated in a primary care provider (PCP) office setting.[10] Increased use of ACSC ED visits has been directly associated with both inadequate EPSDT/well-child care utilization by Medicaid-insured children and by lack of a regular medical home by low-income children.[11] These characteristics may reflect lack of awareness by low-income parents of the availability of EPSDT and its beneficial effects on the physical, social, and cognitive development of children.[12]

History

The Children's Bureau

The history of well-child care in America began with publicly recognizing the need to identify the causes for and methods to prevent maternal and child mortality. With this issue in mind, President Theodore Roosevelt called a conference in Washington, DC, in 1909, subsequently referred to as the first White House Conference on Children.[13] A significant recommendation from this conference was for the establishment of a federal Children's Bureau. After much debate in Congress, President William Howard Taft approved and signed the Children's Bureau into law on April 9, 1912.[14]

The mission for this bureau was "to investigate and report on all matters pertaining to the welfare of children and child life among all classes of our people."[15] Bureau staff initiated studies to identify the social and economic factors contributing to maternal and child morbidity and mortality in both rural and urban settings. The bureau also initiated the routine registration of all births nationwide and the publication of guidelines regarding appropriate prenatal and infant care; these guidelines were presented at professional meetings and were made available to the public.

The Sheppard-Towner Act and the Academy of Pediatrics

Early Children's Bureau findings led to yet another pivotal congressional action strongly endorsed by the newly established contingency of women voters. This action was known as the first Maternity and Infancy Act (or the Sheppard-Towner Act) of 1921.[16] The act provided maternal and child health services, such as maternal outreach education and support through pregnancy and postpartum, as well as instruction regarding parenting and child-health needs. These activities were funded through federal grants-in-aid and matching state funds. With these monies, so-called Sheppard-Towner clinics were established in all but three states (Connecticut, Illinois, and Massachusetts), where opposition was strongest to government-sponsored support for the health of mothers and children. During the congressional debates preceding approval of the Sheppard-Towner Act, many larger cities launched maternal and child health (MCH) activities on their own. Although with this legislation the concept of public responsibility for child health was established, just as today, there was much uneasiness and opposition to the concept of government-sponsored health care. Actual outcome data assessing the effectiveness of these maternal and child clinics were unavailable, but enactment was carried on the "face validity" of their likely benefit.[17] Those opposed to federal grants-in-aid for maternal and child health ultimately won, and in 1929, the Sheppard-Towner Act was not continued.

The physician contingency supporting the Sheppard-Towner Act[18] drove the formation of the American Academy of Pediatrics. In a section meeting of the 1922 American Medical Association (AMA) in St. Louis on diseases of children, the section recognized that the act promoted the welfare of mothers and children, and it elected to approve the Sheppard-Towner Act. However, at the same AMA meeting, the House of Delegates viewed this act as an infringement on the entrepreneurial boundaries of practicing physicians, declared it to be little more than a "socialistic scheme," and reprimanded the section's action. The discord created by this controversy ultimately resulted in the establishment of the AAP in June 1930, which was primarily composed of physicians in favor of the Sheppard-Towner Act. At its founding, the AAP's stated mission was education, public health, and issues affecting child health.

The Children's Bureau, with increased power from the Sheppard-Towner Act, was able to establish well-child clinics throughout rural America and to firmly establish the societal mind-set that there is need for government support for the maintenance of good health (preventive care) from birth through the preschool years. Indeed, the benefit of appropriate dietary and sleep habits for child health was established by the bureau as a health-care paradigm, as was the need for well-child care to facilitate normal development.

Dr. Borden Veeder, author of *Preventive Pediatrics* (1926) and professor of pediatrics at Washington University, predicted that Sheppard-Towner clinics would be replaced by preventive-care physicians (pediatricians).[19] In other words, he predicted that well-child care would become the primary component of some future practices. Between 1928 and 1935, it was reported that approximately 40 percent of pediatric office visits were for well-child or preventive care rather than acute health-care needs.[20] Thus the mind-set of physicians (pediatricians) routinely providing preventive care for children was clearly established by 1935.

Medicaid's Role: Historical and Present

Medicaid was enacted in 1965 as an open-ended, individual entitlement program for eligible children. Shortly after initiation, it was apparent that to be more effective in improving the health status of children, Medicaid needed to have its scope broadened from predominantly acute medical care to include preventive care. In 1967, two years later, Medicaid added the early and periodic screening, diagnosis, and treatment (EPSDT) benefit for children.[21] The primary goal of this benefit was and continues today to be to prevent disease and detect and correct conditions early so that more serious health problems and costly health-care services can be avoided. This preventive-care benefit was designed to ensure that children receive not only care for acute and chronic medical problems but also needed well-child care, including screening, developmental assessment, and immunizations.[22] Unlike the circumstance in Europe, EPSDT is

America's only individual entitlement program for comprehensive health-care services for children.[23]

EPSDT is an entitlement, and federal law requires that states provide the services of EPSDT to all eligible children up to age twenty-one. These services include age-appropriate screenings and immunizations, follow-up diagnostic services for conditions identified in the screenings, and any medically necessary treatment services. Specifically, this preventive-care program provides physical and developmental examinations, vision and hearing screening, dental referrals and treatment, appropriate laboratory tests, and immunizations.[24]

When established in 1967, EPSDT had several problems with implementation at the federal, state, and local levels.[25] Social-science analyses used to evaluate these issues indicated the problems were related to both program design and lack of commitment by state officials to the EPSDT mission.[26] Adjustments were instituted when possible. After this somewhat tumultuous beginning in the 1960s and 1970s, the EPSDT benefit then evolved into a genuine national policy issue between 1985 and 1997. With all but hyperinflationary increases in Medicaid costs, state officials became fixated on Medicaid reform, specifically on changes in the EPSDT benefit that (to them) appeared to represent an unfunded federal mandate placing unnecessary strain on state budgets.[27]

From 1985 through 1997, the congressional debate over the value of EPSDT as a Medicaid benefit for children spun around two groups of powerful policy makers of different thinking regarding this child-health policy. The first group consisted of child advocates, and the second was made up of conservative governors. Though there were additional stakeholders in the issue, such as the White House, Congress, and Medicaid advocates, these two groups were the key participants during two decades of EPSDT political turmoil.[28]

Between 1984 and 1989, increases in Medicaid eligibility for women and children were enacted yearly.[29] Child-advocacy groups such as the Children's Defense Fund, the House Select Committee on Children, the National Committee on Infant Mortality, and Youth and Families supported these enactments.

The acts were also supported by organizations such as the Institute of Medicine and had bipartisan congressional support.

Confrontation and Controversies

The first major EPSDT congressional confrontation occurred in 1989. Despite strong objections from the National Governors Association (NGA), the Omnibus Budget Reconciliation Act of 1989 (OBRA '89) was enacted, making the EPSDT benefit and its preventive-care services federal requirements for all states.[30] The OBRA '89 measures were designed to correct four well-documented weaknesses in the benefit present since its initiation:[31]

1) State establishment of "reasonable standards" for periodicity of well-child examinations
2) State coverage of all medically necessary treatment identified in EPSDT screening
3) State removal of all limitations on participation by any qualified health-care provider
4) State establishment of guidelines to facilitate counting and monitoring all EPSDT patient and provider encounters

States were not enthusiastic about compliance with these OBRA '89 mandates. Discussions of child-health benefits to be included in the design of a national health-care reform bill failed to include stakeholders from several conservative states.[32] This was particularly disturbing for several Republican governors between 1989 and 1994 because they perceived the costs for EPSDT benefits as representing federal infringements on state autonomy.[33]

In designing the Clinton Health Security Plan, EPSDT and other Medicaid benefits for children rapidly became intensely debated policy issues. From 1991 to 1996, Medicaid reform was the primary thrust for the NGA as Medicaid costs consumed larger and larger amounts of state budget dollars. The 1994 congressional elections experienced a shift in congressional control to the Republican Party, which was taken as an opportunity to initiate policy change by the NGA. With the primary goal of balancing the budget, entitlement spending such as Medicaid was a congressional focus. A Medicaid reform bill combining reduced spending with a Republican governors' proposal to reduce federal Medicaid requirements was generated in Congress under the heading "Medicaid Block Grant." This proposal was designed to cap federal Medicaid spending and to give states the power to modify Medicaid regulations.[34]

As an entitlement, Medicaid, like Medicare, guarantees coverage of all eligible individuals. Each state sets its eligibility requirements, but all individuals meeting these requirements are eligible for services. However, each state must pay its share of the federal/state matching funds to receive the federal share. In contrast, federal block grant funding means there is a cap or limit to the federal funds provided each year; under capped funding, a state receives the federal allotment regardless of the level of need or cost. The lack of a guarantee or entitlement to eligible individuals means that with block grant funding, each state can limit the number of people served by using priority lists or even by shutting down programs. Thus, although the use of block grant funding offers states much better predictability of costs for prospective budget planning, it simultaneously allows limitation of service provision to eligible individuals.[35]

All stakeholders advocating for Medicaid as an entitlement program did not have an equal desire to preserve benefits such as EPSDT. In fact, the common element among EPSDT advocates was opposition to the creation of Medicaid as a block grant program.[36] The primary member in this group included Families USA, but the coalition included religious groups, senior citizen organizations, and nursing home and hospital associations. Thus the opposition to the Medicaid block grant proposal was broad and included individuals of all ages that would or could be adversely affected by ending Medicaid as an individual entitlement. The primary goal of this group was to counter the block grant proposal, and the drive to maintain federal guarantees for comprehensive preventive-care services for children was important only to certain groups in the coalition, such as the National Association of Children's Hospitals.[37]

After much wrangling, a pure block grant proposal was generated and passed by Congress to replace the Medicaid entitlement program.[38] This called for a reversal of coverage for many children, and the proposal actually did away with the EPSDT Medicaid benefit. On December 6, 1995, President Clinton vetoed this legislation.[39]

Although the veto was a close encounter for both sides, the anti–block grant forces only narrowly avoided a catastrophic Medicaid policy change in Congress. The NGA was aware of this and set out to generate a new and bipartisan coalition of governors, addressing issues both sides agreed infringed on state autonomy. Although conservative governors saw EPSDT as a drain on their state budgets, they were even more concerned with the specific federal requirements associated with this benefit. Democratic governors most wanted a continuation of Medicaid as an entitlement and continuation of the federal-state Medicaid-funding mechanism. Thus the EPSDT benefit became a bargaining chip for both groups.[40] The issues were considered by a six-member panel of governors, three Republican and three Democratic. This panel then presented its proposal to the full NGA membership and received approval in February 1996.

NGA leaders quickly presented the new proposal to congressional policy makers. A congressional vote called for either the repeal or the redefinition of the treatment portion of EPSDT.[41] The idea was to permit states not to cover all treatments needed by Medicaid-insured children. It included continued Medicaid eligibility for pregnant women and children to age six in families with incomes up to 133 percent of the poverty level, and for children up to age thirteen in families with incomes at or below poverty. The proposal did not include older children.

As this proposal was being debated, a second means of budget reform was also considered. Almost all Medicaid-enrolled children were living in families that qualified for Aid to Families with Dependent Children (AFDC). Thus, separating welfare and Medicaid into two separate budget reform issues could circumvent the current Medicaid debate.[42] Both programs represented areas of large federal spending, and reform in either one would help balance the budget. President Clinton was unwilling to support a Medicaid block grant, but he was willing to accept a welfare reform bill.

State Children's Health-Insurance Programs

The Medicaid issue was for the moment set aside to get welfare reform legislation passed in the form of the Deficit Reduction Act of 1996. This move assured no Medicaid block grant legislation would occur in the 104th congressional session, but the issue was not forgotten. In the next session of Congress, the Balanced Budget Act (BBA) of 1997 gave the NGA almost all that it had been seeking.[43] This enactment included a new State Children's Health Insurance Program (SCHIP) funded as federal entitlement programs to each state by federal block grants. These programs allowed states to mandate enrollment in Medicaid-managed care and to contract with a variety of managed care organizations without a federal waiver. Similarly, guarantees of health coverage for children and at least a partial removal of some EPSDT requirements were included. Entitlement versus block grant funding and the comprehensive EPSDT benefit services were dealt with by increasing eligibility for children in the SCHIPs and permitting each state to decide whether to establish SCHIPs with or without the EPSDT benefit, using purely block grant funding or continuing the current Medicaid entitlement program with EPSDT.[44]

Child health insurance was important to most Americans, and this thinking facilitated passage of SCHIP legislation as a component of the BBA. This program was a large federal commitment to health-insurance coverage for children.[45] Under this new law, states could increase Medicaid or otherwise provide coverage to children whose family income was below 200 percent of the federal poverty level. Unlike Medicaid, which is an individual entitlement to eligible individuals (children and adults), SCHIP was created as an entitlement to states. Further, states were given much authority regarding defining the benefits provided. Thus, two different options were available to each state: Medicaid entitlement versus a new block grant program. The NGA and the AAP supported the proposal based on its likelihood of passage with bipartisan support. Other policy makers favored a Medicaid expansion, including individual entitlements and the EPSDT benefit; this group argued that Medicaid expansion would mean using an existing infrastructure, and with larger numbers of enrollees, the health-care purchasing power would be increased, perhaps with lower cost.[46]

Although many worked to demonstrate the value of a comprehensive child-health benefit, they could not resist the strong opposition to the OBRA '89 EPSDT federal requirements.[47] The final outcome did address the concerns of both sides. The failure by EPSDT supporters reflected the shift in political power and thinking following the 1994 elections. These advocates, however, were able to maintain the federal entitlement to Medicaid and were pleased with the increased government-subsidized health insurance to children coming secondary to increased eligibility. They could not require that the comprehensive Medicaid EPSDT/well-child benefit be a component of SCHIPs—in other words, though EPSDT continues today to be the preventive-care benefit for children insured by Medicaid as a federal-state entitlement program, it is not the benefit used for the new state-designed children's health-insurance programs, which are block grant funded.

Health insurance for children rather than health benefits for children pushed through the 1997 Balanced Budget Act legislation. The majority of Americans supported increased health-insurance coverage but did not support a mandatory, comprehensive well-child benefit.[48]

Future Health-Care Needs

On entering the twenty-first century, the mind-set of public responsibility for maternal and child health, established with the initiation of the Children's Bureau in 1912 and the Sheppard-Towner Act in 1921, remains a frequently debated issue today. For children, Medicaid and the comprehensive Medicaid EPSDT/well-child benefit has only survived with modifications after prolonged and intense congressional debate and passage of the Balanced Budget Act of 1997. Public health insurance for children today includes both Medicaid and SCHIPs; these programs provide insurance to many children beyond those enrolled in Medicaid. SCHIPs are funded as a federal-state block grant, allowing improved state budgetary predictability. The programs do not have the mandatory Medicaid EPSDT/well-child benefit and do not represent individual entitlements.

Today's federal indebtedness requires health-care reform by legislators with prioritization of government-supported health-care services for children and adults. Future expenditures should address the concerns of groups favoring and opposing each budgetary issue. The debate over health care for children—clearly our nation's most valuable natural resource—will undoubtedly continue, with future provisions currently uncertain. However, the need for both availability and access to comprehensive preventive care services, as recommended by the AAP for all children, appears prudent. Simultaneously, the national sentiment regarding governmental support for needed maternal and child health care (established in 1912 with the founding of the Children's Bureau), with the awareness that how the challenges of child health are addressed today will determine our nation's future, remains controversial.[49]

CHAPTER 2

Continuity of Care

*Paul M. Darden, MD, and
William B. Pittard III, MD, PhD, MPH*

Introduction

Continuity of care, a medical home for patients, and primary care are aspects of health care associated with enhanced quality of patient care. In fact, Christakis has suggested that the value of continuity of care is such that it should not be viewed as a process but rather as a desirable outcome to be achieved.[50] The terms "medical home" and "primary care" are concepts that are understood and agreed upon if not consistently operationalized.[51] Much of the discussion of continuity of care has involved the medical home, and continuity of care is considered a key component of the medical home.[52]

This chapter first provides a definition for continuity of care and the medical home, followed by a discussion of the Institute of Medicine's 1994 method for defining quality health care. It then discusses how having a medical home enhances quality and explores what care is like without continuity. Well-child care and continuity are discussed, and studies of both continuity of care and well-child care clinical effectiveness are reviewed.

Continuity of Care and Medical Home Defined

The American Academy of Family Practice (AAFP) defines continuity of care as a process in which the patient and provider are cooperatively involved in ongoing health-care management toward the goal of high-quality, cost-effective medical care.[53] The American Academy of Pediatrics (AAP) defines the medical home as one that provides care to infants, children, and adolescents and that is accessible, continuous, comprehensive, family-centered, coordinated, compassionate, and culturally effective. Explicitly noted in the AAP defined services that a medical home should provide are continuity, acute and chronic preventive care, and needed immunizations.[54] The absence of continuity can lead to fragmentation of care, resulting in a failure to deliver necessary care or the overutilization of resources.[55] The medical home with continuity of care is associated with the delivery of appropriate care, including immunizations.[56] Medical homes offer a solution to care fragmentation.[57] As compared to other avenues of health-care delivery, the medical home is equipped to achieve complete and timely primary care.[58]

Institute of Medicine (IOM) Defines Quality of Care

Although continuity of care has been reported to facilitate the quality of health care, methods to measure the quality of health care are unclear. The IOM, a component of the National Academy of Sciences, Washington, DC, convened a national roundtable on health-care quality in 1994 to bring together a wide variety of well-informed individuals to engage in a series of discussions about health-care quality.[59] Following lengthy interaction regarding health care and cost, it was determined that a national focus on improving the quality of health care was imperative. Specific conclusions reached include the following points:

1) Quality of health care can be precisely defined.
2) While at its best, health care in the United States is superb, often care is not at its best, resulting in identified health-care quality problems in all delivery systems and financing mechanisms.
3) Although a few health plans, hospitals, and integrated delivery systems were noted to have made impressive efforts to improve the quality of care, there were no data indicating components of the health-care system that uniformly and consistently delivered care of the highest

quality, and there was no clear role model of an exemplary delivery system.
4) The roundtable findings indicated a need for effective methodology to improve and monitor the quality of medical care in conjunction with rethinking and reengineering health-care service delivery.[60]

The roundtable endorsed the IOM's earlier definition of quality of care. This 1990 definition was that quality of care is "the degree to which health services for individuals and populations increase the likelihood of desired health outcomes and are consistent with current professional knowledge."[61] The roundtable concluded that quality of care for a great variety of specific clinical conditions and procedures can be measured with sufficient precision to make judgments and to take needed actions to bring about improvement. Either processes or outcomes may be used as valid measures of health-care quality.[62] For an outcome to be a valid measure, it must be closely related to a process of care that can be modified to affect the outcome. For a process to be a valid measure, it must be closely related to an outcome about which the patient cares.

Health-care quality problems were classified by the roundtable into three categories.

1) Underuse—The failure to provide health-care services when they would likely have produced favorable patient outcomes (i.e., failure to detect and treat hypertension or depression, failure to immunize children, prenatal care begun too late in pregnancy, and failure to use effective treatments such as beta-blockers, aspirin, and angiotensin-converting enzyme for all patients who would benefit from these interventions).
2) Overuse—Occurs when a health-care service is provided under circumstances in which its potential for harm exceeds the possible benefit. The RAND Health Services Utilization Study, which now is almost thirty years old,

represents the largest study of health-service overuse ever reported.[63]

3) Misuse—Occurs when an appropriate service is selected, but preventable consequences occur and the patient does not receive the full potential benefit of the service.

This classification of health-care quality problems highlights the relationship between quality and cost of care. Reducing overuse improves quality by reducing unnecessary patient risk and reducing cost. Correcting misuse problems also improves quality by reducing the number of complications and by decreasing cost required to treat complications. Correcting underuse nearly always results in both improved quality and increased cost. This relationship occurs from the fact that, except for immunizations and prenatal care, correcting health-care service underuse generally does not save money. If the service use corrected is effective, improved health status should be identifiable, reflecting increased quality of care, but increased service utilization tends to be associated with increased cost. These descriptions clearly identify the most effective methods to assess the value of health-care services or to determine the health benefit per dollar spent. The largest improvements in value occur when the service increases the value in the numerator of the health status and cost ratio while decreasing the value in the denominator. If we improve the quality by fixing overuse or misuse problems, we have the desired effect on value. The impact on value of correcting underuse of services is less clear because both the numerator and the denominator of the ratio often increase.

The fact that our health-care system faces serious quality problems does not indicate an inadequacy of the skills or motivation of those who provide health-care services. Most problems in health-care quality involve shortcomings in the complex system in which health care is delivered. The strategies proposed by the IOM roundtable to adjust the quality of health-care delivery include the implementation of continuous quality improvement and marketplace competition and improvement incentives. Clearly, the impact of identified health-care quality problems on public health requires alterations from the routine by all stakeholders; meeting this challenge requires a readiness to think in new and different ways about how health-care services are delivered.

The Medical Home Enhances Quality

There is evidence that a longitudinal relationship with a single health-care provider (continuity of care) does enhance the quality of care for patients. Indeed, early brain and cognitive developmental investigation has highlighted the importance of daily routine in promoting optimal personal and social child development.[64] Caregivers who work together are likely to share similar though not identical philosophies regarding primary care practice. Their styles of communication and thinking regarding the importance of attention and responsiveness to children are also frequently similar.[65] This common mind-set provides an environment within which primary caregiving works well for children. The relationships established with primary caregivers in such a setting result in increased health-care satisfaction by the child, the parent, the provider, and the entire caregiving team. All of this represents the underlying principle of continuity of care. Specifically, continuity of care means that children and caregivers remain together for an extended period of time, including at least the first years of infancy.

Keeping children and caregivers together in a familiar setting has several benefits beyond the consistency of a regular primary caregiver:

1) Children also learn to relate in special ways to the other children who share their primary care provider.
2) Continuity of care provides a secure teacher-child relationship and attachment, allowing the provider to develop meaningful rapport over time by becoming quite familiar with the unique needs, skills, interests, and methods of learning of children as individuals.
3) Children develop social skills, including empathy, associated with spending time with the primary care team and fellow patients. Indeed, the likelihood of a child being

socially withdrawn and aggressive with peers has been associated with a lack of a consistent primary caregiver.[66]
4) Within this relationship, parents are more likely to share their concerns regarding their children and listen and comply with the teacher's suggestions.

Thus continuity of care facilitates a provider's ability to generate and put in place health care that will promote a child's immediate developmental needs, and more long-term will enhance readiness for school and life success more effectively than the occasional visit for acute medical care.

Continuity of care appears to be applicable to most health-care systems. Data have demonstrated that several challenges facing US children—from increased school dropout rates, to rising rates of crime, to increasing health-care costs, to competing in the global marketplace—can only be effectively met by addressing the developmental needs of children beginning at birth.[67] Continuity of care is the cornerstone of primary care, is consistent with quality patient care, and helps providers gain their patients' and parents' confidence, enabling the providers themselves to be more effective and empathetic patient advocates. This approach to care facilitates the provider's ability to serve as a cost-effective coordinator of patient health-service utilization through early recognition of problems.[68] Continuity of care is clearly rooted in a long-term patient-provider partnership in which the physician familiar with the patient's history from past exposure can integrate new information and circumstances from the patient's perspective. Continuity of care is facilitated by a physician-led team approach to health care. The AAFP and the AAP encourage primary care providers to promote continuity of care for their patients in all settings.[69]

Continuity of care is certainly consistent with quality care,[70] and this approach incorporates two key perspectives. First, for the family, continuity of care is exposure to a continuous, caring relationship with an identified and trusted health-care provider and team. For providers, the continuity of care ideal is delivery of quality primary care through efficiency, integration, coordination, and the sharing of information with necessary providers. In today's health-care system, patient health-care needs, particularly for patients with chronic conditions, can rarely be completely met by a single professional.[71] However, multidimensional models of continuity of care have been established to accommodate the possibility of receiving care from both a consistent single primary care provider and (as necessary) from a provider colleague or from referral to a specialist, consistently maintaining comprehensive patient history and care understanding by each provider involved.

Continuity is often reflected and assessed by monitoring patient satisfaction with both the interpersonal aspects of care and the coordination of that care within the practice and with necessary referral providers. Experiencing continuity of care is valued by patients in its own right, but this health-care approach clearly facilitates case management as well as multidisciplinary team care. From a provider's perspective, the focus of continuity of care is on service delivery and improved patient outcomes.

Evidence confirms improved health-care quality with continuity of care. These findings include patient and parent satisfaction, physician and staff satisfaction, increased health-maintenance visits, increased immunization rates, fewer sick visits, increased compliance with appointments and medications, increased physician recognition and discussion of emotional and behavioral problems, decreased emergency department visits, and fewer laboratory and imaging studies.[72] Just as continuity of care is associated with increased well-child preventive care as well as general health-care utilization, both well-child care and continuity of care are associated with lower medical care cost.[73] In fact, distinction between the effects of continuity of care and well-child care, which tend to occur simultaneously, is often difficult.

Manifestations of Care without Continuity

To further support the idea of the benefits of continuity of care, we can look at early work in the development of regional immunization registries. These registries indicated that approximately 5 percent of children receive at least one unnecessary immunization by two years of age;[74] this has been termed extraimmunization or overvaccination.[75] Though the use of some combination vaccines can result in acceptable extraimmunization, missing information regarding previous vaccine status can lead to additional extraimmunization as a result of appropriate efforts by medical providers to assure a child's up-to-date immunization status. Extraimmunization may better reflect medical care fragmentation than underimmunization. The latter can also reflect parental choice and lack of access on top of fragmentation of medical care. Thus extraimmunization may serve as a clinical indicator and may, along with other clinical indicators, serve a purpose in testing claims that for a given population of patients, they are actually receiving care in a medical home setting, and that for a given medical home, it is truly eliminating fragmentation of care.[76]

Well-Child Care, Continuity of Care, and Quality: Studies

Although well-child care is the main source of preventive health care for children, and the AAP recommends a widely accepted national standard of frequent well-child visits in the preschool years, compliance with these recommendations by both privately insured and low-income children has been inadequate.[77] Clearly receipt of the AAP recommended well-child care as well as other medical services at a consistent location and from a regular and trusted provider constitutes continuity of care for children, and this care is routinely provided with medical home enrollment.[78] Children with access to a continuous source of care are more likely to receive the full complement of recommended well-child care than those with no medical home.[79] It is therefore difficult to distinguish the effects of well-child care from those of continuity of care. Investigation has demonstrated that continuity of care in infancy is more likely when children receive primary care in a medical home setting.

Simultaneously, children receiving continuity of care are more likely to have health insurance and be up-to-date on their immunizations, and they are less likely to use emergency department (ED) services.[80] At the same time, the anticipatory guidance component of well-child care has been long recognized as the foundation for health-care supervision and preventive care for children.[81] Though the visits are perhaps more likely to occur with a continuous relationship between caregiver and patient, receipt of the AAP-recommended well-child visits in the first two years of life has been associated with both reduced ambulatory care sensitive condition (ACSC) emergency department (ED) visits birth to six years and school readiness at the conclusion of the five-year kindergarten (K–5) school year.[82]

Lastly, to determine whether compliance with the recommended well-child care schedule independent of continuity of care is associated with variation in the rate of ACSC hospitalizations, an additional study assessed children under the age of four years (n = 36,944) with and without chronic illnesses.[83] In this study, continuity of care was assessed using the continuity of care index as described by Bice and Boxerman.[84] These children were retrospectively monitored for adherence to the recommended well-child care schedule and for their access to continuity of care. The children with and without chronic disease with low well-child care adherence and low continuity of care were both found to be associated with increased risk of ACSC hospitalization in the first four years of life. Thus, this analysis suggests that lack of a consistent source of primary care and inadequate well-child care are both associated with increased risk for ACSC hospitalization by children. Separation of the effects of continuity of care from those of well-child care is at best difficult.

Conclusion

Although continuity of care and well-child care are quite different components of primary care, their individual benefits to children overlap, are synergistic, and are quite difficult to distinguish. Caregivers for children take on the large responsibility of meeting the primary care and health-education needs of a relatively small number of the larger population of parents and children. The caregiver, through continuity of care, can provide a consistent and genuine, personal relationship with children and their families that in and of itself facilitates physical and social development. Simultaneously, as a component of primary care, the caregiver encourages utilization of the AAP-recommended well-child care, which is also designed to promote optimal physical and social development in children. Just as anxiety is anticipated for children with the annual transition between teachers in the school setting, and as specific efforts are frequently made to reduce this stress (such as having children visit their new class and new teacher or having the new teacher visit the child in his or her class prior to the transition), similar strategies have been suggested to reduce primary-care stress when clinicians change. These continuity of care procedures in the school setting are intended to reduce ineffective learning, and continuity of care in clinical practice is intended to facilitate the patient-provider relationship with an enhanced quality of care.

Continuity of care represents a core component of quality health care for children. Children learn and develop more readily when they are in a secure, trusting, and familiar setting. Children are more satisfied with care and are able to develop both physically and socially with a trusting caregiver relationship. Certainly such relationships offer the foundation for early exploration and learning by children, facilitating successful long-term development.

CHAPTER 3

Well-Child Care Screening

James R. Roberts, MD, MPH
Kristina K. Gustafson, MD, MS

Introduction

Primary care providers conduct various screening procedures throughout childhood, beginning in the newborn period and continuing through adolescence at all well-child visits. Many screening procedures are routine enough to be considered universal, but others such as lead screening and tuberculosis testing, once universal, are now conducted on children considered at greater risk. This chapter explores the well-child screening procedures conducted in the first six years of life as recommended by the American Academy of Pediatrics (AAP), and it discusses the tangible benefits provided.

The goal for screening procedures is to detect disorders that are serious or even life threatening, for which there are available treatments to reduce complications or even prevent disease. With screening, disease detection and treatment can occur before outward signs and symptoms (clinical symptomatology) are even apparent—and for some disorders, before outcomes become irreversible. Some illnesses that are screened for are rare, and false positive screenings may be a source of parental anxiety. However, with screening procedures, the early detection and treatment of rare but devastating disease is possible.

Newborn Screening for Metabolic and Other Conditions

The newborn screening program in each state is actually well-child care conducted in the hospital newborn nursery setting. The

American Academy of Pediatrics (AAP) recommends that the first well-child visit occur in the primary care provider's (PCP's) office at about one to four weeks of age;[85] this visit is crucial for assessing the results of the newborn screen. States frequently send newborn screening results to the hospital where a child was born or to the physician provider group responsible for the child's care in the newborn nursery. Of course, the child may present to a second physician or physician group for well-child care. Nevertheless, the PCP to whom the child presents must ensure that the results of the newborn screening are assessed and reviewed with the parents.

Definition of Related Conditions

Newborn screening represents procedures for testing all newborns for the presence of disorders that are harmful or even fatal but that are not apparent upon physical examination at birth. Many of these disorders are metabolic, and therefore this testing is often referred to as the newborn screen for inborn errors of metabolism, although other diseases are also screened for in this system. The metabolic disorders most commonly screened for tend to be those that profoundly alter a specific process in the body (i.e., energy production, waste disposal, or toxin deactivation). Metabolic screening began in the 1960s with assessment for phenylketonuria (PKU) and has today evolved into a battery of several different metabolic diseases, including galactosemia, medium-chain acyl-CoA dehydrogenase deficiency (MCAD deficiency), homocystinuria, and maple syrup urine disease (MSUD).

Endocrine diseases are also included in many state newborn-screening panels, including congenital hypothyroidism (CH) and adrenal hyperplasia (CAH). Newborn screening can also detect homozygous hemoglobin SS disease (the most common form of sickle cell anemia). This screening panel may also identify the "C" hemoglobin, which when combined with hemoglobin "S" will present phenotypically as sickle cell disease (Hgb SC disease), although generally this disorder is less severe than that of hemoglobin SS disease. Although rare, if identified early, these disorders can be effectively treated with normal or significantly improved mental and physical outcomes.

Many disorders can be screened for with less than one drop of blood using mass spectrometry, but the federal government does not mandate which particular disorders each state must include in screening programs. Therefore, the disorders screened for vary from state to state. The decision as to which disorders are actually tested for is set by each state health department based on a cost-to-benefit ratio. The cost involves more than simply the dollar amount for a procedure and includes the risk of false positive testing (sensitivity and positive predictability of the procedure) and the availability of treatments for the disorder. A list of the diseases that are commonly screened for is shown in table 1.

Table 1. Most common diseases in newborn screening programs and their specific tests

Condition	Type of Test	Comments
Congenital hypothyroidism	Thyroid stimulating hormone (TSH)	Increase in false positives first 48 hours
Congenital adrenal hyperplasia	21-hydroxylase accounts for 95% of CAH	Increase in false positives before 24 hours
Sickle cell anemia	Hemoglobin electrophoresis	Detects hgb S and C
Galactosemia	Classic: (Galactose-1-phosphate uridyl transferase) Type II (Galactokinase def)	Classic: jaundice, FTT, vomiting, liver failure, bleeding, sepsis. Type II is less severe, usually only causes cataracts

Biotinidase deficiency	Biotinidase	Seizures, hypotonia, hearing loss, ataxia, developmental delay Immediate and lifelong treatment with biotin prevents all effects
Phenylketonuria (PKU)	Phenylalanine (levels are increased)	Defect in the enzyme phenylalanine hydroxylase
Citrullinemia type I	Argininosuccinate synthetase	Disorder of urea cycle Ammonia and other toxic substances build up in blood
Medium-chain acyl-coenzyme A dehydrogenase (MCAD) deficiency	Tandem mass spectrometry MCAD profile demonstrates elevated levels of medium chain acylcarnitines	Other disorders of fatty acid oxidation have been added in many other states
Tyrosinemia	Tyrosine (elevated levels)	Defect in tyrosine degradation, which generates the toxic (and diagnostic) metabolite succinylacetone
Homocystinuria	Methionine	Abnormal amino acid metabolism Elevated homocysteine levels

| Maple syrup urine disease | Leucine and valine are both elevated | Defect in the enzyme branched chain ketoacid dehydrogenase Abnormal amino acid metabolism |

Benefits of Screening

Early recognition of CH and PKU has prevented significant mental retardation in children. In both cases, once the developmental and neurological effects from the disease are present, they are irreversible. Recognizing the various enzyme abnormalities in CAH, particularly in boys because there are no genital abnormalities as in girls, has been lifesaving.[86] If undetected in the newborn period, CH will cause severe developmental delay within three to four months, and these effects are frequently irreversible. Although female infants with CAH tend to present with the physical findings of virilization, male infants with CAH frequently have a normal physical exam and will only present with severe and potentially life-threatening salt-wasting crisis around three weeks of age.

For the other commonly screened for disorders in table 1, early identification can prevent serious disability and death if identified and treated early. Though these are uncommon disorders, they fit several important characteristics of disease for which a screening procedure is well designed: they are detectable before clinical symptomatology is present, there is an available treatment, and the treatment may improve or correct the disorder.

Hearing Screening

Definition of Related Conditions

Hearing loss can be categorized as conductive, sensorineural, or central. Conductive and sensorineural hearing loss can occur together. Conductive hearing loss occurs when the structures that mechanically convert sound (including the tympanic membranes and ossicles) are damaged, usually from recurrent or persistent otitis media. Sensorineural hearing loss occurs when structures that transduce sound waves into nerve impulses are damaged, including the cochlea and auditory nerve. Central hearing loss is characterized by a deficit in the brainstem or processing centers in the brain. Hearing loss is also classified as congenital or acquired. The congenital hearing loss is often sensorineural, but there are some conductive forms of congenital hearing loss.

Procedure

Infants are screened in the first twenty-four hours of life in most US hospitals; in the event of a home delivery, the infant should have a screening within the first month of life.[87] There are two tests that can be used in the newborn period: the evoked otoacoustic emission (OAE) testing and the auditory brainstem response (ABR). The OAE sends clicks or tones to the infant's ear and then detects sound from the cochlea. The ABR measures electroencephalographic waves from the vestibule-cochlear nerve. False positives may be more common using the OAE, which can be affected by middle-ear debris, a common issue following cesarean delivery. Repeat screening using the ABR may be effective in reducing false positives. If ABR is not available in the newborn nursery, referral to an audiologist should be done before three months of age.

Follow-up for all newborns who fail hearing screening should be strongly encouraged by PCPs because it has been reported that the follow-up rate is approximately 76 percent in one large study.[88] Similar to the follow-up for the newborn screening at the one-week well-child visit, the results of the hearing screen should be assessed by the PCP in the first postdischarge well-child visit.

Young children who need to be screened but are not able to be tested with simple audiometry screening in the office should be referred to an audiologist. This referral should be done when otitis media is clinically suspected, especially to assess children with chronic otitis media.[89]

Well-Child Care in Infancy

Epidemiology of Related Conditions

The incidence of congenital hearing loss is about one to three per one thousand live births.[90] This is a more common congenital illness than any of the others screened for as part of the battery of newborn screening. Most acquired hearing loss is conductive, and the most common cause of conductive hearing loss is chronic or persistent otitis media with effusion.[91]

Benefits

Infants in a newborn screening program receive early diagnoses and referral and treatment compared to those who are not screened.[92] This early identification of CHL can greatly enhance normal child development, particularly receptive and expressive language. Based on the available evidence following hearing screening implementation, the US Preventive Task Force (USPTF) has concluded that hospitals should offer this service.[93] The earlier a patient with a sensorineural hearing loss is referred, the greater the likelihood that definitive treatments such as cochlear implants will be effective. Children even younger (less than two years) outperformed all other age groups.[94] A second study conducted in the Netherlands evaluated the developmental outcome of children at three to five years of age. Those who were screened in the newborn period and were found to have hearing loss performed better on developmental testing compared to those children who were identified at a later date using distraction hearing assessments.[95]

In early childhood, much of hearing loss may be caused by recurrent otitis media with effusion, and the effect and progression of hearing loss may be more subtle. Many children may be in the range of mild to moderate hearing loss, and as such they may not even be detected without having a hearing screen. The benefit of identifying mild acquired hearing loss and subsequent draining of middle ear fluid is controversial and depends on the outcome measure in question.[96] Most other studies, including several from well-designed, randomized control trials, have failed to show an improvement in neurodevelopmental hearing loss at follow-up through nine to eleven years of age.[97]

Vision Screening

Definition of Related Conditions

All infants and children need to have an eye examination and an assessment of visual acuity as early as possible. Though standard visual acuity screening in the primary care setting requires a cooperative child looking at a chart, an ophthalmologist can assess acuity at an earlier age. The key is conducting an appropriate physical examination to identify infants who need to be referred.

Specific terms used in discussing visual screening include

- strabismus, which is the misalignment of the eye;
- pseudostrabismus, which is the appearance of misalignment of the eyes due to some other facial structure, usually prominence of the inner epicanthal folds; and
- amblyopia, which is the loss of visual acuity due to cortical suppression.

Strabismus is a major cause of amblyopia, and the physical findings of strabismus should indicate to the PCP that the child has or is at risk for having amblyopia.

Procedure

Visual screening begins in the newborn period with examination of the external eye structures. Persistent discharge or tearing should be noted. Ptosis of one or both eyelids may cause amblyopia and should also raise the suspicion for other neurological abnormalities. The eyes should be equal in size and shape. The pupils should be of equal size and should be equally reactive to light. An assessment of the red reflex should be done, and the presence of a white reflex or absent, dull, or otherwise abnormal appearance should be referred to an ophthalmologist.

Infants and Toddlers

All physical assessments included in the newborn examination should be repeated at subsequent well-child visits. Failure to fixate after three months should be a cause for an ophthalmology referral.

Children Three Years and Older

All of the previous assessments should be performed annually. In addition, after three years, a formal vision assessment should be attempted using a standardized vision screening tool. For children older than four, a chart with Snellen letters may be used instead of the pictures and symbols charts. If the child is not yet cooperative beginning at the age of three, he or she should be reexamined in six months. Abnormal findings on visual acuity assessment include twenty-fifty at age three, twenty-forty at age four, and twenty-thirty on or after age five.[98]

Epidemiology of Related Conditions

Approximately 5–10 percent of preschool children will have some type of vision problem, including amblyopia, strabismus, and refractive error. Four percent of preschoolers will have strabismus, and of those with strabismus, 40 percent will have related amblyopia. Prior to the AAP recommendations for vision screening in pediatric practice in 1986, half of the children with amblyopia and strabismus were not diagnosed before age five.[99]

Benefits

Recognition of decreased visual acuity can be corrected with glasses or contact lenses. Unfortunately, if children fail a vision screen either in the office or another setting such as school, there is a risk that they may not go to a specialty eye care provider, and those who do may not have good compliance in terms of wearing their prescribed corrective lenses.[100] One study evaluated a comprehensive follow-up program for children that failed on a school vision screening; this clinical trial provided free eye examinations and free glasses at the time of the screening. Although more expensive, this procedure did not have a striking impact on compliance by children.[101]

Identifying conditions such as strabismus (which may eventually result in amblyopia) and initiating appropriate therapy can improve the strabismus and perhaps limit or prevent the loss of visual acuity. In a longitudinal study of vision screening in children at or less than three years of age, a one-time screening at thirty-seven months resulted in a decrease in the prevalence of amblyopia by 60 percent. Early screening was even better, with a 70 percent decrease in residual amblyopia when screening was started at less than three years of age.

The earlier that patients with amblyopia and related conditions that can lead to amblyopia are identified, the better the outcome that follows. One case-control study compared seventy-five children with late diagnosis (five years or greater) to eighty-six children who were diagnosed at an earlier age. When controlling for socioeconomic status and family experience with similar disorders, early diagnosis of strabismus led to earlier identification of amblyopia along with correction of the disorder. Children who had the diagnosis of strabismus were more likely to have been seen by a PCP who did not consistently use the appropriate newborn examination techniques, including red reflex identification and an evaluation of extraocular motility to identify strabismus in infancy.[102]

A review of the US Preventive Task Force (USPTF) has established a recommendation for universal vision screening between ages three and five years based on the available evidence that early treatment of amblyopia improves outcome. Though clinicians continue to conduct vision screening in the form of physical examination techniques, the USPTF has concluded there is inadequate evidence that vision screens less than three years of age will improve visual acuity.[103]

Developmental Screening

Definition of Related Conditions

Children undergo major developmental changes with regard to motor, communication and language, cognitive, and social-emotional skills during the first six years of life. At well-child visits, an individual child's development is assessed to determine if the observed development differs from similar aged norms. If a child is not progressing at the appropriate pace or following the expected sequence of skill emergence as peers, or if the child displays a regression in skills, providers should assess the child further for this developmental irregularity.

Two types of developmental assessment occur during well-child visits. Developmental surveillance is the process by which PCPs watch for signs of developmental or behavioral problems to identify children at risk for developmental delay. In contrast, developmental screening includes use of brief standardized tools to identify children who do or do not need more extensive evaluation.

In 2006, the AAP revised its policy statement to include a detailed developmental screening algorithm in an effort to guide PCPs on how and when developmental surveillance and screening should occur.[104] After the 2006 AAP revised policy statement and in a follow-up survey of AAP members, Radecki and colleagues found that pediatricians' use of standardized screening tools increased significantly from 2002 to 2009, especially with reference to the use of the ages and stages questionnaire and the parents' evaluation of developmental status.[105]

Procedure

As of 2001, the AAP recommended that all children should receive standardized developmental screening as part of well-child care. According to the AAP, children should be monitored at every well-child visit by the pediatrician using developmental surveillance.[106]

The algorithm for developmental surveillance and screening includes ten steps:

1) Have the pediatric patient come to a preventive care visit.
2) Perform surveillance.
3) Does surveillance demonstrate risk?
4) Is this a nine-, eighteen-, or thirty-month visit?
5) Administer screening tool.
6) Are the screening tool results positive or concerning?
7) Make referrals for developmental and medical evaluations and early developmental intervention or early childhood services.
8) Developmental and medical evaluations.
9) Is a developmental disorder identified?
10) Is child identified to have special health-care or chronic-condition management needs?[107]

All concerns with language and communication before three years of age should stimulate the PCP to consider early identification, audiology, and speech-language pathology referrals, especially if they are persistent at an early return visit.

There are numerous categories of developmental screening tools available to identify a wide spectrum of disorders. According to Marks and LaRosa, the most commonly used broadband screen for children in the first six years of life include the ages and stages questionnaire and parents' evaluation of developmental status.[108]

Epidemiology of Related Conditions

Approximately 1–3 percent of all US children have some form of developmental delay.[109] Detection rates for developmental delay are lower than the actual prevalence. Isolated developmental delay of one or more domains is fairly common. Approximately 25 percent of cases of developmental delay have an identifiable underlying etiology.[110] The likelihood of identifying the underlying etiology is higher in children with global developmental and motor delays (greater than 50 percent) compared to children with isolated language disorders (less than 5 percent).[111]

Benefits

Identifying developmental delay allows PCPs to know which children need referrals for support, such as physical, occupational, or speech therapy. More important, early communication skills including eye contact, orienting to name, or pointing can be assessed, and early intervention can be initiated in the first year of life if there is a pathological delay. For example, early correction of hearing deficits has been found to enhance associated developmental delays. Early intervention strategies are available for speech and language as well as motor disorders, and they have been found effective.[112]

Autism Screening

Definition of Related Conditions

The term "autism" represents a group of conditions that are referred to as autism spectrum disorders (ASDs). ASDs are a group of neurologic disorders that are characterized by impairment in social interactions and communication skills. Signs of autism such as subtle deficits in social skills or preverbal gestural language can be noted in most effected children by eighteen months of age. PCPs focus on four DSM-IV criteria to help identify children younger than three years of age that might have an ASD.[113] The four DSM-IV criteria that are applied to children under three years include delayed expressive language development, impaired use of nonverbal behaviors (including a lack of social or emotional reciprocity with caregiver or others), a preoccupation with stereotyped and restricted patterns of interest, and lack of joint attention. The last item is a behavior necessary for functional language development, in which the infant shows enjoyment with sharing an object or event with another person by looking back and forth between the two. Physicians can also rely on prompting by parents who voice a concern about absent or delayed speech.[114] The majority of parents become concerned between fifteen and eighteen months of age.[115] Lack of speech has been considered a hallmark of autism.

Procedure

According to the AAP, all children should universally have the autism-specific screening tool administered at the eighteen-month well-child visit.[116] This autism-specific screening tool should be obtained in addition to the general developmental screening tool that is also administered at that time. The most commonly used tool is the modified checklist for autism in toddlers, or M-CHAT.[117] Details about the components of this tool and other standardized instruments are beyond the scope of this chapter. However, a second screening with the autism-specific screening tool should be done at the twenty-four-month well-child visit and at any encounter where the parent voices a concern.[118]

Epidemiology of Related Conditions

According to the Centers for Disease Control and Prevention's Autism and Developmental Disabilities Monitoring (ADDM) Network, the estimated prevalence of autism spectrum disorders has been increasing.[119] In 2000 and 2002, the incidence of ASDs was approximately 6.7 per 1000 children, or about 1 in 150 children. This estimate was 8.0 per 1000 children (1 in 125) in 2004 and 9.0 per 1000 children (1 in 110) in 2006. Data from 2008 reveals an ASD incidence of 11.3 per 1000 children (1 in 88).

ASDs occur in all racial, ethnic, and socioeconomic groups. The CDC's ADDM notes that ASDs are 4.6 times more common in boys (1 in 54) than in girls (1 in 252). Genetics appears to play a role in autism spectrum disorders. Advanced parental age has been associated with increased risk of having children with ASD, perhaps due to de novo spontaneous mutations or genetic imprinting alterations. It has been reported that compared to the general population, parents having one child with an ASD are at increased risk for having a second affected child. Among identical twins where one child has an ASD, the other child is affected 36–95 percent of the time, and approximately 10 percent of children with autism also have genetic or chromosomal conditions such as down syndrome, Fragile X, or tuberous sclerosis.[120] ASDs frequently occur with other developmental, neurologic, and psychiatric disorders, and more than 80 percent of children with an ASD diagnosis also have another developmental disorder diagnosis.

Benefits

There are positive benefits of developmental and behavioral interventions for children who have ASDs, especially when it is initiated before the child is three years of age. Thus, early diagnosis (before age two) is beneficial; this will facilitate a timely referral to early intervention services, which has the potential to improve language and social development as well as function in educational settings.[121] The primary screening tool, the M-CHAT, has a positive predictive value for identifying ASDs early in childhood.[122] Early diagnosis is also helpful for younger siblings of children diagnosed with an ASD because they are ten times more likely to have an ASD than children in the general public.[123] Access to intervention services at an early age may provide better prognostic outcomes in certain children with ASDs. These programs promote development of communication, social, adaptive, behavioral, and academic skills.[124]

Lead Poisoning Screening

Definition of Related Condition

Lead poisoning was originally diagnosed based on observable clinical symptomatology, including mental status changes, coma, seizures, and often severe anemia. Over time, abnormal subclinical findings have been documented in children with blood lead levels (BLLs) once considered normal. This has led to changes in the definition of lead poisoning to BLLs that adversely affect children's development, behavior, or cognitive development but in which outward clinical signs or symptoms are not necessarily apparent.

The first published statement by the CDC in 1975 indicated that a blood lead level of less than 30 mcg/dL was "normal." Blood lead levels greater than 30 mcg/dL are associated with clinically evident signs and symptoms, including abnormal pain, constipation, or even mental status changes and seizures.[125] In subsequent statements, the CDC altered its terminology and grouped children based on their BLL into classes I, II, III, and IV, with class I being the lowest risk of symptomatology and class IV having the greatest risk with BLL greater than 70 mcg/dL.[126] Lead is a heavy metal that has no physiologic purpose in the human body, and so there is actually no such thing as a "normal" BLL. The CDC appropriately removed the word "normal" from subsequent statements regarding BLLs and eventually used the term "action level."

Research in the 1970s through the early 1990s noted subclinical effects, including loss of IQ points among children with BLLs between 10 mcg/dL and 25 mcg/dL, as well as inattention and hyperactivity.[127] Thus the CDC action level has been gradually lowered with interim levels of 25 mcg/dL in the 1980s to 10 mcg/dL in 1991.[128] Subsequent research demonstrated that much of the subclinical effects occurred in children with BLL below 10 mcg/dL.[129]

This research subsequently led to a statement released by the CDC in 2012 that eliminates the use of the phrase "level of concern" and instead focuses on the approximately 450,000 children whose blood lead concentration falls at or below the 97.5 percentile on the distribution of BLL in one- to five-year-old children in the National Health and Nutrition Examination Survey (NHANES). Children at or above this reference value of 5 mcg/dL must undergo monitoring of their BLL. The CDC also reinforced their emphasis on the role of primary prevention.[130]

Procedure

Screening for lead poisoning in children today is initiated with a questionnaire to determine risk. Primary risk factors include residing in a home built before 1950, ethnicity, and low family income. Childhood lead poisoning is best determined using a blood lead level (BLL), which can be accomplished either using a capillary sample (finger stick) or a venipuncture. Capillary samples are valid as a screening tool, but if elevated above the action level as set by the CDC (currently 5 mcg/dL), a venipuncture must be obtained for confirmation.[131]

As a proxy for household income, the CDC recommended that children who are Medicaid-insured should be screened with a BLL regardless of the answers on the lead questionnaire.[132] Given that parents of children enrolled in Medicaid may be renting their home and therefore may not know the age of their home, parental responses regarding home age may not be a reliable assessment of lead risk.[133] When in doubt, a BLL should be considered.

Epidemiology of Related Conditions

The prevalence of lead poisoning, as measured by an elevated BLL (using the previous lead action level of 10 mcg/dL), has shown a steady decline in the past two decades. Data from the US National and Nutrition Examination Survey (NHANES) from the early 1990s demonstrated a prevalence of 4.4 percent.[134] Follow-up NHANES data from 1999 to 2002 found a prevalence of 1.6 percent.[135] Data from the same source in 2004 found a further decline in the US prevalence of lead poisoning to 1.4 percent.[136] The prevalence of lead poisoning and indeed of BLLs in general is highly dependent on the age and condition of housing in which individuals live. Therefore, communities with a high percentage of homes built before 1950 are associated with increased risk for lead poisoning.[137] Likewise, lead poisoning is more likely to occur in minority children and in children with lower family incomes. Since the most recent change in the CDC reference value to 5 mcg/dL, there has been no data generated indicating the prevalence of elevated BLL (EBLL) at this level of concern. However, it should be noted that with the skewed distribution of elevated blood lead levels, comparisons of the prevalence of lead poisoning between EBBL of 5 mcg/dL and 10 mcg/dL is difficult to accurately assess. More research needs to be done regarding improving the use of data from screening programs.[138]

Benefits

There is little doubt that screening for lead poisoning has had a significant impact on the health of children in the past forty years. Until the late 1970s and early 1980s, it was commonplace for children to have serious, even life-threatening, acute lead encephalopathy with seizures, coma, and death.[139] Chelation for lead poisoning was once a regular reason for childhood hospitalization, with numerous reports of severely lead-poisoned children frequently published in the 1950s and 1960s.[140]

The initial goal of the early blood lead screening programs was to attempt to identify children before they were symptomatic and prevent their BLLs from rising to a level often associated with seizures and acute encephalopathy. One of the earliest lead screening programs in the United States was conducted using door-to-door screening in Charleston, South Carolina. Researchers noted that 32 percent of the children had a BLL greater than 30 mcg/dl.[141] National screening for lead poisoning became a focus for the CDC in 1975, enabling more children to be identified prior to clinical symptomatology. The severe acute lead encephalopathy noted in the 1950s and 1960s became less common.

The CDC changed the action level to less than 10 mcg/dL in 1991, which shifted the emphasis to identifying children at high risk for lead poisoning before they became symptomatic.[142] The approach to targeted screening in 1997 based on age of housing and children's epidemiological risk factors further cemented efforts to selectively screen.[143] The change in risk-based screening has enabled identification of thousands of children who may have behavioral and cognitive deficits due to BLL in the 10–30 mcg/dL range who would have never been identified before, because there were no clinical signs of lead poisoning. Both screening and subsequent emphasis on primary prevention have played major roles in reducing the national prevalence to its current levels of 1.6 percent.[144]

Today, child hospital admissions for chelation is the exception rather than being routine, and though it was once a disease

Well-Child Care in Infancy

process with serious morbidity and mortality, lead poisoning as a public health problem has been significantly reduced in the past two decades.[145] Children are now identified earlier and before any clinical symptoms are evident. Fewer children have elevated BLLs on the national level,[146] and families are much more aware of lead poisoning, particularly in communities where children have been previously affected by lead.[147]

Iron Deficiency Screening

Definition of Related Conditions

Iron deficiency (ID) refers to the iron stores in the body, and iron deficiency anemia (IDA) refers to an abnormally low hemoglobin concentration caused by iron deficiency. Although they are often referred to collectively as iron deficiency, it is important to recognize that children may be iron deficient without being anemic. With this understanding, because the initial screening test is designed to detect iron deficiency anemia, the CDC and most PCPs consider a hemoglobin level under 11.0 g/dL in children between twelve and thirty-five months of age as the cut point for IDA, although a total iron level is required to diagnose IDA. Iron deficiency without anemia is defined as having insufficient iron stores to maintain normal physiologic functions.

Procedure

The AAP recommends universal screening for IDA by obtaining a hemoglobin level at the age of one year; this sample may be obtained via finger stick. Hemoglobin (Hgb) levels can and should be measured in older children who have additional risk factors present for iron deficiency, including feeding problems, poor growth, and a dietary history of inadequate iron intake.[148] Although not considered part of the standard universal screening recommendations of the AAP, children with socioeconomic risk factors are also often screened for IDA at two years, usually coinciding with a second blood lead level determination.

William B. Pittard III, MD, PhD, MPH

Epidemiology of Related Conditions

According to the 1999–2002 NHANES data, the US prevalence of iron deficiency and IDA was 9.2 percent and 2.1 percent, respectively. The prevalence in the United States varies widely based on race, ethnicity, and family income. Mexican Americans have the greatest proportion of toddlers with ID and IDA. The prevalence of children enrolled in the women, infant, and children service (WIC) was greater than the general population as well (ID of 10.7 percent and IDA of 3.1 percent). The prevalence was slightly higher in non-Hispanic white (7.3 percent ID and 2.0 percent IDA) versus black (6.6 percent and 1.6 percent).[149] With the variation in ID and IDA in WIC and Medicaid-enrolled children, it is likely that PCPs that care for a high percentage of children enrolled in these programs are more likely to have a significant burden of ID and IDA in their practices compared to providers that care for more affluent children. A clear association exists between iron deficiency and cognitive and behavioral functional delay, and although most criteria to assume causality have been at least partially satisfied, there remains insufficient data to conclude that ID with or without anemia causes cognitive delay.[150]

Benefits

Screening children for iron deficiency allows early and appropriate doses of supplemental iron to be prescribed to correct both ID and IDA. Despite long-term use of the hemoglobin screen in young children, there are only a few blinded studies to evaluate whether correcting the anemia improves cognitive development in children less than two years of age. Most short-term trials have too few participants or were randomized with a control group to determine whether iron replacement facilitates cognitive function. Children in these studies demonstrate that at follow-up, those whose hemoglobin was corrected to normal continued to demonstrate cognitive delay. Therefore, it is not clear how cognitive dysfunction is actually related to iron deficiency, although the anemia can be corrected with therapy. This subject has been summarized in several publications.[151]

Tuberculin Skin Testing

Definition of Related Conditions

Tuberculosis (TB) is a treatable disease caused by infection with mycobacterium tuberculosis, a complex organism that actually represents a group of acid-fast bacilli (AFB) including *M. tuberculosis*, *M. bovis*, and *M. africanum*. Most M. tuberculosis complex infections in children and adolescents are asymptomatic, thus making it important for providers to determine which patients need to be screened. When the disease does occur, the clinical manifestations often appear one to six months after the initial infection. *M tuberculosis* complex is transmitted via inhalation of airborne droplets from a contagious adolescent or adult who has laryngeal or pulmonary TB. Children are often infected by exposure to these contagious individuals and are asymptomatic. It is imperative to identify infected children because they can be treated, thus preventing the perpetuation of the disease and its complications. For a more detailed clinical description, see the AAP Committee on Infectious Diseases, Red Book.[152]

A child with no signs or symptoms of disease is determined to have latent tuberculosis infection if he or she has a positive tuberculin skin test (TST) and a chest radiograph that is normal or has calcifications suggesting a healed infection. If a young child develops latent tuberculosis infection, it suggests that there was a recent transmission, which may help in determining the source case.

Procedure

The AAP and the Pediatric Tuberculosis Collaborative Group have recommended a selective medical screening approach[153] that involves a risk assessment; if positive, a screening using the TST should be performed. The risk assessment includes questions regarding contact with a tuberculosis case, regular contact with high-risk adults, and birth in or travel to high-risk countries. This questionnaire has been found to have adequate sensitivity and specificity when compared with the presence of a positive TST.[154] The questionnaire should be first completed by age one month. The provider should inquire again at the six-, twelve-, and eighteen-month well-child visits, and then annually starting at two years of age.

According to the AAP, CDC, and the American Thoracic Society, the only reliable TST method is the intradermal injection of tuberculin purified protein derivative (PPD) by the Mantoux method.[155] The Mantoux method consists of 5 tuberculin units of PPD (0.1 mL) injected intradermally using a 27-gauge needle and a 1.0 mL syringe into the volar aspect of the forearm.[156] Creation of a palpable induration 6–10 mm in diameter is essential to accurate testing. After placement of the TST, the amount of induration (erythema without induration should not be included in the measurement) in millimeters should be assessed forty-eight to seventy-two hours later. A positive test is one of three measurements of induration including at least 5 mm, at least 10 mm, or at least 15 mm based on the patient's tuberculosis risk factors as determined via the risk-factors questionnaires.[157]

Epidemiology of Related Conditions

Currently, the prevalence of TB in US children is at a historic low. Over a ten-year period, the CDC documented that 60 percent of all counties had no pediatric cases of TB, with only twenty-five counties in urban settings reporting more than one hundred cases.[158] Tuberculosis occurs in all ages, and the rates are higher in urban, low-income communities. Eight out of ten cases in the United States occur in nonwhite and Hispanic individuals. More than 25 percent of newly diagnosed cases in children less than fourteen years of age are diagnosed in foreign-born children. The populations with greatest rates of latent (asymptomatic disease) and symptomatic tuberculosis infection include the homeless, residents of correctional facilities, immigrants, international adoptees, and refugees from or travelers to high-prevalence areas such as Asia, Africa, and countries of the former Soviet Union. Among overseas travelers and members of the military, the cumulative incidence is 2 percent.[159]

Benefits

When asymptomatic infection (latent tuberculosis) is identified via targeted screening, treatment can be initiated. Screening also identifies the disease earlier and prevents spreading. Some states (or counties within states) still recommend universal screening. However, selective screening with a questionnaire and then subsequent TST, if needed, is more cost-effective than universal screening.[160] Even with targeted screening in areas with low prevalence, considerable cost and high rates of false positive testing are problematic.[161]

Blood Pressure Screening

Definition of Related Condition

Recent findings indicate that many common and costly adult chronic health conditions such as obesity, hypertension, dyslipidemia, diabetes mellitus (DM), and metabolic syndrome have their origins in childhood.[162] Elevated blood pressure (BP) as a child is a risk factor for early adult hypertension, which in turn is a risk factor for other cardiovascular disorders. As such, the PCP can serve an important role in addressing the developmental precursors of these adult cardiovascular problems. Due to this, the National High Blood Pressure Education Program Working Group on High Blood Pressure in Children and Adolescents made recommendations regarding screening and management of pediatric hypertension in 2004;[163] they defined hypertension for children as an average systolic or diastolic BP greater than the ninety-fifth percentile for gender, age, and height on more than three separate occasions. Prehypertension is an average systolic or diastolic BP that is greater than the ninetieth percentile but less than the ninety-fifth percentile. Like an adult, adolescents with a BP greater than 120/80 mmHg are considered prehypertensive.

Procedure

A blood pressure measurement is a noninvasive, cost-effective, and generally accurate method to identify pediatric hypertension. According to the Expert Panel on Integrated Guidelines for Cardiovascular Health and Risk Reduction in Children and Adolescents, it is recommended that children less than three years of age with specific conditions identified below have selective BP screening.[164] Reasons for which children in this age group should be screened include the following:

1) A history of prematurity, very low birth weight (<1500 grams) or other neonatal complication requiring intensive care
2) Congenital heart disease, regardless of operative status
3) Recurrent urinary tract infections, hematuria, or proteinuria
4) Known renal disease or urologic malformations
5) Family medical history of congenital renal disease
6) Solid organ transplant
7) Malignancy or bone marrow transplant
8) Treatment with medications known to elevate blood pressure
9) Other systemic illnesses associated with hypertension, such as tuberous sclerosis, neurofibromatosis, etc.
10) Evidence of elevated intracranial pressure

In 2004, the National Heart, Lung, and Blood Institute (NHLBI) recommended that providers assess blood pressure in all children starting at three years of age at every medical encounter.[165] In 2011, an NHLBI task force recommended annual blood pressure measurement in children over three years of age,[166] and the AAP and Bright Futures Handbook endorsed this recommendation.[167]

Epidemiology of Related Conditions

Hypertension occurs in 2–5 percent of US children; however, the incidence appears to be increasing.[168] Based on epidemiologic surveys over the past twenty years, the incidence of BP has been increasing in children, as has the prevalence of hypertension and prehypertension explained partially by the increased incidence of obesity.[169] Prehypertension progresses to hypertension at a rate of approximately 7 percent per year. Approximately 33 percent of boys and 25 percent of girls continue to have hypertension in a two-year longitudinal follow-up study. The increased prevalence of obesity coupled with high calorie and salt intake and physical inactivity most likely contribute to this trend.[170]

Benefits

Despite recommendations of the NHLBI and their endorsement by the AAP, the US Preventive Task Force (USPTF) does not endorse a specific recommendation regarding blood pressure monitoring in children due to inconclusive evidence.[171] Additional studies are needed to better assess the risk of childhood hypertension and subsequent development of secondary cardiovascular disease as adults. Though the harm from universal blood pressure screening is low, the US Preventive Task Force has not determined that the benefits outweigh any harm.

Several studies suggest that although childhood blood pressure screening has not been shown to impact long-term health outcomes, early identification of hypertension may facilitate the health status of some who are at risk for cardiovascular disease as adults. Hypertension (HTN) in children may predict HTN in adults.

A prospective cohort study of 2,445 children compared BP measurements in children (between seven and eighteen years of age) and again in young adulthood (twenty to thirty years of age). Children with BP greater than the ninetieth percentile were 2.4 times more likely to have BP greater than the ninetieth percentile as adults than those with lower BP in childhood. Most children (94 percent) with at least three normal BP readings had normal BP readings as adults. Additional evidence has been published exploring the association between childhood and adult BP.[172]

Some evidence has also suggested that elevated BP in childhood is related to secondary cardiovascular changes as adults. A retrospective study assessed records from children aged ten to seventeen who were admitted for elective surgery and compared their BP at the time of surgery with their adult outcomes regarding coronary artery disease (CAD). There was no association found between childhood BP and CAD. Of note, children with BP greater than the ninety-fifth percentile were four times more likely to have CAD than children with BP below the ninety-fifth percentile.[173] Children with uncontrolled essential hypertension experienced increased cardiovascular load with resulting left ventricular hypertrophy (LVH) in 40 percent of children with hypertension.[174] Unfortunately, there is no evidence that treating HTN in childhood reduces adult cardiovascular complications.

Body Mass Index Screening

Definition of Related Conditions

Body mass index (BMI) is a tool used to identify children who are overweight or obese. Children are categorized as overweight and obese based on their measured body mass index (BMI). The BMI is based on the child's height measured in meters, with the weight measured in kilograms (BMI = wt/ht^2; weight in kilograms, height in meters). Obesity is defined as a BMI greater than the ninety-fifth percentile, and overweight is defined as a BMI between the eighty-fifth and ninety-fifth percentile for children of the same age and sex.[175] BMI does not directly measure body fat, but it is or can be a helpful indicator of adiposity. A child's weight status is determined by multiple factors, including genetics, metabolism, nutrition, physical activity, and environment. A balance between healthy eating habits and regular exercise is a key parameter to maintaining a healthy weight during childhood.

Numerous health effects are related to childhood obesity. Obese children can have CAD, left ventricular hypertrophy, hypercholesterolemia, dyslipidemia, hepatic steatosis, insulin resistance, and metabolic syndrome. They also are at increased risk for asthma and obstructive sleep apnea, as well as social stigma, depression, and loss of self-esteem.

Procedure

A child's BMI was first recommended to determine overweight and obesity in 1991.[176] The AAP has published recommendations for management of childhood overweight that include early (beginning at two years) and ongoing screening and tracking of BMI percentiles.[177] The BMI is plotted against age and sex percentiles to determine the BMI percentiles using CDC growth charts for children two to nineteen years old, which are available from the CDC (http://www.cdc.gov/growthcharts/clinical_charts.htm). They recommend the PCP encourage healthy nutrition and physical activity behaviors.[178]

Epidemiology of Related Conditions

In the past twenty-four years, the prevalence of both childhood overweight and obesity has more than doubled. Children who are either overweight or obese can have pulmonary, orthopedic, GI, neurologic, cardiovascular, and endocrine health consequences. Children who are overweight have a higher prevalence of high blood pressure, increased blood lipid levels, impaired glucose tolerance, and insulin resistance. Overweight adolescents are now more frequently plagued with the "adult morbidity" of type two diabetes mellitus, which had been previously uncommon in childhood. According to NHANES III, 31 percent of overweight children aged ten to sixteen years were diagnosed with asthma as compared to 14.5 percent of children whose BMI was under the eighty-fifth percentile. Using the same study data, 6.8 percent of overweight and 28.7 percent of obese children qualified as having metabolic syndrome (hypertension, hypertriglyceridemia, low HDL cholesterol, and hyperinsulinemia) as compared to 0.1 percent of normal weight children (BMI under the eighty-fifth percentile).

The prevalence of pediatric obesity has increased worldwide, with developed countries experiencing a more rapid rate of increase than developing countries. Despite intense clinical focus on management of the "obesity epidemic" in children, the rates have only plateaued and have not actually declined.

Approximately 17 percent of children in the United States aged two to nineteen are categorized as obese by the CDC.[179]

Childhood obesity has numerous secondary related conditions. Hypertension and DM type II are almost three times higher in the obese pediatric population. Children with obesity are more likely to have elevated blood pressure and high cholesterol levels. These are risk factors for cardiovascular disease (CVD). In one study, 70 percent of obese children had at least one CVD risk factor, with 39 percent having two or more.[180] Obese children are at increased risk of type two diabetes as a result of increased risk for impaired glucose tolerance and insulin resistance.[181] Children with obesity are at risk for fatty liver disease and gallstones.[182] The prevalence of asthma and sleep apnea with childhood obesity is 31 percent and 6.8 percent, respectively.[183]

Benefits

Obese children are more likely to become obese adults and more severely obese as adults.[184] Adult obesity is associated with serious health problems.[185] Early identification of patients with obesity can lead to a multistep approach to help slow or stop weight gain, or to possibly reduce weight. Children should be encouraged to increase physical activity while decreasing high-calorie and low-nutrition foods. Many patients are more likely to reduce their weight in a peer health group with others who can relate more effectively. With achievement of a normal BMI, the risk of complications from obesity does return to that of the normal weight of the general population.

Conclusions

Primary care providers perform many screening procedures throughout the first six years of life. All provide substantial benefits to the health and well-being of childhood, although they do vary somewhat in the level of disease prevention. These benefits don't quite reach the level of protection or the historical lifesavings that vaccinations to infectious diseases have provided; however, the role of screening is different from vaccinations. Vaccinations are the reason why polio is an exceedingly rare event, and why the prevalence of Haemophilus influenza meningitis is dramatically lower. Nonetheless, the benefits for AAP-recommended early childhood screening programs allow for early detection of numerous disease processes or disorders; they achieve a level of secondary prevention in order to detect a problem early so that changes in health-care delivery or public health practices can be initiated. In some cases, the disorder can be identified before there are any outward clinical signs or symptoms, such as in lead poisoning, tuberculosis, or hypertension. In other situations, early detection of the disorder or disease allows for interventions to be put into place before significant effects or irreversible damage occurs, such as in hearing loss, vision loss, and metabolic disorders.

CHAPTER 4

Well-Child Care Parental Anticipatory Guidance in the Preschool Years: Clinical Effectiveness

William B. Pittard III, MD, PhD, MPH

Introduction

Child health as measured by infant mortality continuously improved for American children throughout the second half of the twentieth century, in conjunction with improved acute and preventive medical care.[186] This outcome, however, was less dramatic for low-income as compared to more-affluent children.[187] Indeed, the scenario of inadequate preventive care, poor health, and lack of school readiness is disproportionately shared by low-income children.[188]

This chapter first defines the parameters of well-child care visits. Then it reviews the responses of key stakeholders to the delay in confirming clinical effectiveness for each component of well-child care. How this information gap has influenced well-child care utilization by children and the delivery of this preventive care by providers is noted. Lastly, this chapter describes recent findings regarding the clinical effectiveness of the nonimmunization components of well-child care, or, more specifically, studies showing the association (effectiveness) between parental receipt of well-child anticipatory guidance instruction and both reduced use of hospital emergency departments (EDs) for nonurgent ambulatory care sensitive conditions and school readiness at the conclusion of the five-year kindergarten (K–5) school year.

Well-Child Care Visits

The American Academy of Pediatrics (AAP) recommends a widely accepted national standard of frequent well-child and preventive-care visits in the preschool years, including six in the first year, three in the second, two in the third, and one annually thereafter through age twenty years.[189] The Medicaid well-child benefit is called early and periodic screening, diagnosis, and treatment (EPSDT) and includes, as recommended by the AAP, parental anticipatory guidance, screening procedures, and immunizations.[190]

The AAP Bright Futures Handbook succinctly describes the content of EPSDT and well-child visits.[191]

- Recommendations for the anticipatory guidance component focus on parental health education, including child nutrition, appropriate health-care utilization, exercise, and cautions regarding child safety and hazards to cognitive development such as iron deficiency and lead exposure.[192]
- Screening or secondary preventive care is recommended to identify the presence of certain diseases as well as disorders in growth, hearing, vision, and cognitive development early enough to initiate corrective therapy, limiting complications and cost.
- Age-appropriate immunizations or primary preventive care is recommended to reduce infectious disease morbidity.

All of these well-child services are intended to result in more extended periods spent without illness, fostering the development of cognitive, linguistic, and social skills via more time spent in play and interaction with other children and adults.[193]

The anticipatory guidance portion of a well-child visit, particularly in the preschool years, informs and reminds parents of safety measures and behavioral characteristics they need to put in place and anticipate in preparation for the developmental stages their children will soon enter.[194] Behavioral changes such as crawling, walking, and climbing, as well as needed safety measures to avoid unintentional injury, are presented to parents on an age-appropriate basis before (if possible) children actually reach each stage. Parental safety measures include avoidance of toxins such as lead or common household chemical products as well as smoke and other adverse exposures.[195] Additional injury prevention topics include protective headgear for bicycle riding, child car seats for vehicle transportation, and needed protective devices for sports activities.[196] Anticipatory guidance also involves review of the child's nutrition status, physical activity and exercise, oral health, television exposure, sleep habits (including positioning), activities to enhance cognitive development such as parent-child reading and writing (coloring), and suggestions to expand social interaction with other children and adults.[197]

All of the recommended topics for anticipatory care would be too time consuming and perhaps unnecessary for every child at each visit. Ergo, anticipatory guidance for different parents and children at different ages requires topic prioritization for individual needs.[198] Although standardization for such an important activity as anticipatory guidance could perhaps prevent topic omissions, it appears unrealistic if for no other reason than the fact that child and family needs are not all the same, even for children of similar ages. Therefore, a quasi-standardized approach to well-child care amenable to change based on provider and parent-perceived need may be more likely to facilitate normal physical, emotional, and cognitive child development than a strictly regimented (standardized) approach.

Both Medicaid and privately insured preschool children use fewer EPSDT and well-child visits than recommended by the AAP.[199] Though inadequate insurance coverage (underinsured) and high co-payments are reported to reduce well-child care utilization by privately insured children, Medicaid-insured children, despite government funding, underuse well-child care more than those privately insured.[200] This fact has been attributed to the health-care-seeking behavior of Medicaid children and their guardians, provider responsiveness to low-income families, and the health-care system itself.[201] Thus, access to preventive care via health-care funding does not ensure utilization of services.[202] The underuse of EPSDT by Medicaid-enrolled preschool children has been associated with poor health, lack of school readiness, and more frequent use of emergency departments (EDs) for nonurgent ambulatory care–sensitive conditions (ACSCs).[203]

Due to a lack of empirical data, the AAP-recommended number and content of EPSDT and well-child visits were originally based on consensus expert opinion.[204] Upon realizing this information gap, in the early 1970s the AAP requested investigation assessing the clinical effectiveness of these recommendations.[205] Three decades later, the effectiveness of well-child care recommendations remained confirmed only for immunizations and some screening procedures. Only in the last six years have data indicating effectiveness of the parental anticipatory guidance component of well-child care been published using quasi-experimental observational studies.[206]

This delay in confirming well-child care effectiveness other than for immunizations has resulted from study experimental design difficulties. Unlike the other components of well-child care, vaccines and immunizations undergo randomized clinical trials confirming safety and effectiveness prior to Federal Drug Administration (FDA) approval and licensing. Thus, the effectiveness of immunizations is empirically established prior to their becoming components of well-child care.

Because it is widely accepted that each component of well-child care promotes the health status of children, randomization of study children into groups to receive and not to receive the AAP-recommended number and composition of EPSDT visits is considered unethical.[207] Therefore, studies assessing effectiveness for the parental anticipatory guidance and screening components of well-child care have used nonrandomized quasi-experimental observational techniques.[208] Using observational methodology, investigators observe outcomes (such as health-care utilization and school readiness) by children that receive at least as many and those that receive fewer than the recommended number of EPSDT visits.

Observational studies can establish a significant association between dependent (outcome) variables and independent variables (such as receipt of the recommended EPSDT and well-child visits), but due to lack of randomization, they cannot establish that the outcome observed was caused by the independent variable.[209] Also, to avoid selection bias due to lack of randomization, associations between outcomes observed (health-care utilization and school readiness) and EPSDT utilization are estimated using regression analyses, adjusting for previously identified confounding factors such as maternal age, education, parity, prenatal-care adequacy, race and ethnicity, family income, and urban or rural residence.[210] An additional limitation with using this methodology to assess well-child care effectiveness is that there is no adjustment in the regression models for innate variation in parenting responsibility.

Clearly, children of responsible parents are more likely to attend preventive-care visits and to have healthy development. Appropriate health-care utilization skills are routinely taught via parental health education as part of the anticipatory guidance component of well-child care. The hypothesis tested in recent studies has been that children who receive the recommended number of EPSDT visits in infancy have improved health status compared to those who receive fewer than the recommended number. Thus, with reference to anticipatory guidance, it is hypothesized that the health status outcomes, including the number of ACSC ED visits and school readiness, will be improved for children who receive the recommended EPSDT visits and whose parents receive the recommended anticipatory guidance health education as compared to children who receive fewer visits and whose parents receive less parental health education.[211]

The long delay in confirming well-child care clinical effectiveness has also been attributed to the observation that the health status of children is much more influenced by poverty and other social factors than by well-child care.[212] Ergo, though the parental anticipatory guidance component of well-child care may contribute to improved health status for children (the outcome), this factor may simply have an effect that is too small to be detected without larger sample sizes than used in many studies.

Well-Child Care Utilization and Lack of Confirmed Clinical Effectiveness

Well-child care utilization reflects input from several stakeholders, including private- and public-insurance administrators, health-care providers, parents, and, to some degree, children themselves. The delay in confirming clinical effectiveness for the parental anticipatory guidance and screening components of well-child care has influenced each of these stakeholders, and these influences have been reflected at least in part by the utilization of this preventive care.[213]

Public- and Private-Insurance Administrators

First, the lack of data confirming well-child care effectiveness in improving the health status of children has influenced public- and private-insurance policy makers. This effect became more pronounced with the publication of findings by the Institute of Medicine (IOM).[214] These IOM findings indicate that although correction of the underuse of needed health-care services increases the quality of care, it also increases cost. Public and private administrators want improved quality of care. However, if the effectiveness is unproven and the cost is likely to increase, the incentive for the introduction of methods to correct the underuse of well-child care is at best limited.[215]

Health-Care Providers

In contrast to insurance administrators, health-care providers have consistently maintained an optimistic perspective regarding the unproven benefits of parental anticipatory guidance.[216] In training, providers are taught that parental health education is designed to promote child health and development. Therefore, the argument that parental health education provides support and family reassurance that is beneficial to child health has strong face validity for providers. These stakeholders, even without empirical evidence, have thus accepted that parental anticipatory guidance is clinically effective and have strongly encouraged its use.[217]

Parents and Children

Parents and their children have a third, somewhat mixed perspective regarding parental anticipatory guidance. Although education and counseling are reassuring and satisfying for many parents, due to limited provider time and cost, this component of well-child care is less satisfying and educational to others.[218] Clearly, children are seldom enthralled with receiving immunizations or most other components of well-child care, although rapport with their primary care provider (PCP) is often quite strong.[219] With today's large number of recommended anticipatory guidance topics and newer health issues for many children, such as obesity, human immunodeficiency viral infection (HIV), behavioral problems, attention-deficit/hyperactivity disorder (ADHD), and depression, providers must prioritize both time and topics necessary to meet the unique needs of both parents and children. This is a task for which providers have often received little training, and it undoubtedly influences satisfaction with and utilization of well-child care.[220]

Impact of Stakeholders

The discrepant thinking regarding the clinical effectiveness of parental anticipatory guidance between parents, health-care providers, and policy makers almost certainly offers some understanding for the reported lack of well-child care utilization by children in the preschool years.[221] The large number of recommended topics to be covered under anticipatory guidance (parental education), the variations in access to care by children, the differences in parental understanding regarding the benefit and cost-effectiveness of well-child care, and the variation in specific approaches taken by PCPs in the provision of anticipatory guidance have stimulated a serious ambivalence regarding preventive care. In today's multicultural society, parents and children require greater individualization of well-child care rather than a more standardized approach, because their needs are more diverse than in the past. These variations require increased utilization of e-mail communication between parents

Well-Child Care in Infancy

and providers and between parents, health-care providers, and other community stakeholders partnering to facilitate the normal growth and development of children.

Parental Anticipatory Guidance and Evidence-Based Medicine

Evidence-based medicine represents recent efforts to guide the safety, effectiveness, and cost of clinical practice using science and social science methodologies in empiric investigation to facilitate more standardized and effective care.[222] Prior to the recognized need for evidence-based medicine, physicians often directed medical care according to their medical training, individual experience, and community custom.[223] Patients and third-party payers, with minimal access to information regarding care options, depended on physicians to provide their best judgment for care. This process has changed dramatically with the recognition of a need for evidence linking findings with recommendations for care.[224]

Historically, when uncertain about the best treatment for a patient, the medical community suggested care that "made sense" or "should work effectively" based on provider clinical experience even when there was little empirical evidence of effectiveness. Unfortunately, when this treatment appeared to have a positive response, PCPs continued to use this approach for similar illnesses and encouraged colleagues to do the same. By default this treatment became a health-care paradigm that continued even after the treatment was found via empirical investigation to not be effective or even to be detrimental.

A similar mind-set or culture has served as the driving force for the provision of the AAP-recommended well-child care. Providers in training are taught, and therefore believe, that the AAP-recommended number and content of well-child visits facilitates optimal growth and development and reduces morbidity and mortality for children.[225] Specifically, the teaching has been

1) that children who receive the AAP-recommended number and content of well-child and EPSDT visits in the first years

of life have less morbidity and mortality and improved physical, emotional, and cognitive development compared to children who receive fewer than the recommended number of visits;
2) that this reduced morbidity is associated with fewer emergency department (ED) visits;
3) that reduced morbidity and ED use reduces long-term health-care cost; and
4) that children with the recommended well-child care are more likely to be ready for school at the conclusion of their K–5 school year.

These outcomes are assumed to be secondary to improved nutrition, reduced illness, improved social interaction with other children and adults, and enhanced parenting behavior as compared to children with fewer visits. With this training, pediatricians and child care providers have consistently argued that the unproven benefits of recommended well-child care are clear, and this thinking has driven their practice. Indeed, their contention has consistently been that lack of empirical evidence should not be construed as lack of effectiveness for well-child care.[226]

Recent findings regarding the clinical effectiveness of parental anticipatory guidance have been generated from a six-year prospective study of a three-year birth cohort (2000–2002) of South Carolina children consistently enrolled in Medicaid throughout the preschool years (birth to two years, n = 36,662, and birth to six years, n = 18,512). A single study in a given community or state usually lacks the diversity of persons, settings, or outcome measures to be considered generalizable to the nation.[227] However, these findings, presented in several different peer-reviewed publications, describe outcomes for Medicaid-insured children cared for and funded under federal guidelines applied to all fifty state Medicaid agencies, providing broad generalizability.

This study generated data for three published reports in 2007, 2011, and 2012.[228] These reports are discussed in the sections below. The outcomes for children receiving all the recommended

EPSDT/well-child visits in year one versus those who did not were reported in 2007. The association between receiving the AAP-recommended visits in the first two years of life and health-service use and school readiness birth through six years for these children were reported in 2011 and 2012, respectively.

EPSDT Visits and Health Outcome

The first study was reported in 2007.[229] This analysis tested the hypothesis that Medicaid-insured children with the AAP-recommended number of EPSDT visits in the first year of life have better health outcomes in the second year than those with fewer visits. The data analyzed represented all health encounters for study children continuously enrolled in a fee-for-service (FFS) Medicaid health-care model birth to twenty-four months (n = 36,662).

To accurately assess the association between well-child care and health-service utilization, a control for baseline child health was established by excluding children with conditions that could predispose them to utilize more well-child care and that would not necessarily be evenly distributed among the children in the EPSDT utilization groups. Excluded children were those with major congenital anomalies, including sickle cell anemia and with recognizable genetic malformations. Study children were also restricted to those who were full-term and appropriately grown at birth, requiring thirty-seven to forty-two weeks gestational age and excluding those with a birth weight less than the fifth or greater than the ninety-fifth percentile for gestational age.[230]

For these analyses, the results were adjusted for maternal and child characteristics, including maternal age, race/ethnicity, family income, education, urban/rural residence, and parity and child gender, gestational age, and birth weight. For each outcome monitored, such as sick-child doctor visits, the rate of utilization was determined for the children with at least and with fewer EPSDT visits than recommended. These data were used to generate a rate ratio where the rate for children with at least the recommended EPSDT visits was the numerator. Rate ratios less than 1.00 suggest that children having at least the recommended number of EPSDT visits had less utilization of the given outcome. For each outcome, the rate ratio estimate was presented with the estimated lower and upper bounds of the ninety-fifth percentile confidence interval (CI).

Associations were first examined between the rate ratios of EPSDT visits in the first year and health-care use in the second year, including sick-child PCP visits, emergency department (ED) visits, hospital admissions, and hospitalizations and ED visits for ambulatory care sensitive conditions (ACSCs). ACSC diagnoses are sick-child illnesses routinely treated in a PCP office. The diagnoses monitored included those reported to be the most common ACSC ED and hospital admission diagnoses for Medicaid children, including asthma; seizures; cellulitis; ear, nose, and throat infections; bacterial pneumonia; kidney and urinary tract infections; and gastrointestinal infections.[231]

Children with at least the recommended number of EPSDT visits in year one had a higher adjusted rate of sick-child (ACSC) PCP visits (rate ratio, 1.49: 95% CI, 1.41–1.58), and a lower adjusted rate of ACSC ED visits (rate ratio, 0.94: 95% CI, 0.89–0.99) in year two than children with fewer than the recommended visits in the first year. Having at least the recommended preventive-care visits was not associated with differences in rates of general ED visits or of hospitalizations. Thus, having at least the recommended number of EPSDT visits in the first year of life was associated with a shift in health care from the ED to the PCP office for ACSC diagnoses in the second year.

Parental Anticipatory Guidance and Long-Term Health-Service Use

A second report from this six-year prospective cohort study was published in 2011. This evaluation tested the hypothesis that Medicaid children with the recommended EPSDT visits in the first twenty-four months utilize fewer ACSC ED services and more ACSC PCP visits from birth to six years than children with fewer visits.[232] The data for this analysis included all health encounters for children continuously enrolled in Medicaid from birth to six years (n = 18,512). The study examined the association between receiving the AAP-recommended number of EPSDT visits and utilization of health-care services. Children with the recommended EPSDT visits had a greater adjusted rate of sick-child (ACSC) PCP visits (rate ratio, 1.62: 95% CI 1.50–1.76) and a lower adjusted rate of ACSC ED visits (rate ratio, 0.88: 95% CI, 0.81–0.95). Thus the use of the recommended number of EPSDT visits in infancy was associated with a shift in health care from the ED to the PCP's office setting by Medicaid children throughout the first six years of life.

A plausible explanation for these two observations regarding ACSC ED use and EPSDT utilization in infancy is that mothers of children with at least the recommended number of EPSDT visits receive more child health education regarding health-service utilization via anticipatory guidance, and they perhaps develop a closer provider-parent relationship than mothers of children with fewer visits. Thus, they may be more likely to bring their sick children to the PCP's office, rather than to the ED. This would be a desirable outcome for obtaining the recommended number of EPSDT visits. Indeed, it appears likely that most state Medicaid offices would consider a significant reduction in the occurrence of costly and potentially preventable ACSC ED visits throughout the first six years of life to be a useful manifestation of well-child care clinical effectiveness.

Parental Anticipatory Guidance and School Readiness

Underuse of EPSDT services and lack of readiness for first-grade learning have been reported to disproportionately affect children insured by Medicaid.[233] Inadequate school readiness has been associated with poverty and poor health,[234] a lack of reading material and cognitive stimulation in the home, and cultural variation in beliefs and attitudes about education.[235] A detailed review of the AAP-recommended well-child care content was summarized and published in 2007;[236] this review concluded that the parental anticipatory guidance component of preschool well-child care is designed to promote both the well-being and longer-term school readiness by preschool children.

The third report from the six-year South Carolina prospective cohort study was published in 2012 and tested the association between receipt of the recommended number of well-child visits in the first two years of life and school readiness at the conclusion of the K–5 school year.[237] This observation was that children whose parents received anticipatory guidance instruction as they received the recommended number of EPSDT visits in infancy had 23 percent increased odds of being ready for school (OR, 1.23, 95% CI, 1.10–1.37) as compared to children whose parents received less parental education because they received fewer EPSDT visits.

Parents of children with the recommended number of well-child visits in the first two years of life receive more information via parental anticipatory guidance than others about methods of cognitive stimulation for their children such as reading and writing with them, encouragement in social interaction with other children and adults, and more information and education about avoiding risks to physical and cognitive health such as lead exposure and iron deficiency.[238] Thus one might anticipate that children, whether privately or publicly insured, who have at least the AAP-recommended number of well-child visits in the first two years of life will be more likely to be ready for school at the conclusion of the K–5 school year than those with fewer visits.

Indeed, parents of children with at least the recommended number of EPSDT visits receive more guidance from their child's health-care provider about child health and parenting, whereas their children receive more screening and preventive care than children with fewer visits.[239] Parents or caregivers who receive more guidance about child development and parenting may be more likely to offer their children learning activities in the preschool years. Because they receive regular health education and guidance about risk avoidance, these parents may also improve their child's diets, promote physical activity, arrange more social activity, and avoid environmental toxins, all of which may be associated with improved brain development and the social skills required for school readiness.[240]

Receipt of the recommended number of well-child visits in the first two years of life is associated with a shift in care from the ED to the PCP office for ACSC diagnoses throughout the first six years (and with increased odds for school readiness), and so efforts to improve the utilization of well-child care in infancy appear prudent.[241] Fewer than 10 percent of Medicaid-insured and less than 70 percent of privately insured children receive the recommended number of EPSDT and well-child visits in the first three years of life.[242] Thus the potential to increase these percentages with improved quality of care and possibly increased school readiness is large. Improving school readiness by correcting the underuse of well-child care may be well worth extra cost.[243]

Conclusion

This chapter has reviewed the variation in responses by parents, health-care providers, and both government and private-insurance administrators to the long delay in confirming clinical effectiveness for the individual components of EPSDT and well-child care and how these responses have contributed to the utilization of this comprehensive preventive-care benefit by children. Lastly, the chapter has described the recent findings indicating clinical effectiveness for the parental anticipatory guidance component of EPSDT care.[244]

Two significant associations are described with receipt of the AAP-recommended number of EPSDT and well-child care in the first two years of life, and specifically with the health education from the parental anticipatory guidance component. Both of these associations include enhanced continuity of care and suggest that the effectiveness of well-child care parental anticipatory guidance in the first twenty-four months of life in improving the health status of children extends throughout and perhaps beyond birth to six years.

These observations suggest two findings. First, there is a cost-efficient shift in care from the more expensive ED to the less-expensive PCP office setting for ACSC diagnoses birth to six years by children with the recommended visits as compared to those with fewer visits.[245] This finding indicates that use of the recommended number of EPSDT visits in the first twenty-four months with increased parental health education is associated with more cost-efficient health care throughout the first six years of life. The second observation is that children with the recommended number of EPSDT visits in the first two years of life have greater adjusted odds of being ready for school at the conclusion of the K–5 school year than children with fewer visits.[246] These observations are both consistent with the expectation that parents of children having at least the recommended number of EPSDT visits in the first two years receive more guidance about child health and parenting behavior and that their children have improved general health and cognitive development.

Lack of objective evidence confirming the clinical effectiveness of well-child care, and particularly the nonimmunization components, has resulted in a serious gap in available information. Lacking such evidence, some policy makers have been uncertain whether introducing methods to correct the underuse of well-child care is worth any added short-term cost.[247] The findings discussed in this chapter indicate that receipt of the recommended well-child care—and more specifically the parental anticipatory guidance component—is associated with higher quality care manifest by more cost-efficient service use and increased school readiness. Pending additional research that may support these findings, the implementation of methods to correct the underuse of EPSDT care by Medicaid children appears to be a prudent financial investment.

CHAPTER 5

Routine Immunizations Birth to Six Years: Clinical Effectiveness

Paul M. Darden, MD

Introduction

Immunization and vaccination have profoundly improved children's health, and in the words of Susan and Stanley Plotkin, "The impact of vaccination on the health of the world's people would be hard to exaggerate. With the exception of safe water, no other modality, not even antibiotics, has had such a major effect on mortality reduction and population growth."[248] Immunization is a critical component of preventive care for children. For the first two years of life, the periodicity schedule for well care and the routine immunization schedule are almost identical. As the AAP Bright Futures recommends, throughout childhood routine immunizations should be given as part of well-child care.

Parents, their children, and physicians have seen substantial growth in the number of diseases vaccinated against and changes in the type of vaccines used. From birth to six years, the number of diseases protected against through routine immunization has gone from eight in the late 1950s to thirteen in 2013 (see figures 1–4 below). With this expansion has also come the notable event of the eradication of smallpox from the world and the elimination of the smallpox vaccine from the immunization schedule.[249] Associated with this growth in routine immunization has been a concomitant decrease in diseases of childhood.

This chapter will cover the history of immunization and the immunization schedule, discuss the goals of immunization, present the vaccination schedule, and discuss the effectiveness and economic impacts of vaccination.

History of Immunization and of the Immunization Schedule

It is not clear when vaccination as a deliberate attempt to protect children and adults against diseases began. Indications go back as far as tenth-century China, and medical texts from the eighteenth century outline various means of protecting against smallpox going back to 1695.[250] Smallpox epidemics ravaged Boston throughout the colony's early days. In 1721, a British vessel arrived in Boston Harbor. During the first day, one of the ship's crew was diagnosed with smallpox and quarantined. Soon nine more seamen from the ship were determined to have smallpox, and cases began to appear among Boston residents. As the number of smallpox cases mounted, approximately 1,000 residents fled Boston. Ultimately, 5,980 contracted smallpox, and 844 (14 percent) died before the epidemic subsided. The influential Bostonian Puritan Minister Cotton Mather was a strong proponent of variolation, a view not common among Boston physicians. However, Mather convinced Zebdiel Boylston, a friend and practicing physician, to undertake smallpox vaccination. Although many were saved, Boylston was arrested but later released on the condition that he would not inoculate anyone without government permission.[251]

In the United States, it could be argued that smallpox vaccination was instrumental in winning the Revolutionary War. After a disastrous attempted invasion of Canada beginning in 1775 and followed by a counteroffensive by the British, an epidemic of smallpox ravaged the Continental Army, with over half of the American troops developing smallpox. Subsequently, the Continental Congress authorized Washington to order compulsory smallpox vaccination of every recruit, resulting in an army free of smallpox.[252]

Massachusetts passed the first immunization law in the United States requiring smallpox vaccination for the general population in 1809, and subsequently other states enacted similar legislation. In 1905, the case of *Jacobson vs. Commonwealth of Massachusetts* upheld the constitutionality of compulsory vaccination.[253] State

Well-Child Care in Infancy

and local laws that mandate vaccinations, especially for school entry, have played a substantial role in disease reduction.[254] How these compulsory vaccination laws are formulated and enforced can lead to different degrees of protection for the public.[255]

Types of Vaccines

The first vaccine was commonly used against smallpox. The next vaccines routinely recommended were developed in the twentieth century and were primarily targeted at diseases of childhood. Since the 1960s, recommendations for the immunization of preschool children have been made by the American Academy of Pediatrics (AAP) through its Committee on Infectious Diseases and Advisory Committee on Immunization Practices (ACIP). Beginning in 1995, the AAP, working together with the American Academy of Family Physicians (AAFP), has annually published a harmonized immunization schedule.[256]

In the late 1950s, the recommended vaccines for preschool children were smallpox, polio (as IPV), diphtheria, tetanus, and pertussis (the last three given in combination as DTP). In the late 1960s, vaccines to protect against measles, mumps, and rubella were developed and added to the schedule as the combined vaccine MMR. Also, the inactivated polio vaccine (IPV) was replaced with the oral polio vaccines.[257] MMR and OPV were live virus vaccines. In the 1970s, the smallpox vaccine was eliminated from the schedule with the eradication of the disease in the United States.[258]

The vaccines and the age of administration recommended by the ACIP in 1983[259] are shown in figure 1. In this and all the vaccine schedules presented, the footnotes are key to implementing the vaccine schedule. Only the figure is presented here because it illustrates the vaccines and the timing of the vaccines. If one is interested, the footnotes can be found in the referenced articles. As of 1983, there were two combination vaccines, DTP and MMR, as well as one oral vaccine, OPV. In 1995 (figure 2) with the first harmonized schedule, two additional vaccines were added for preschool children, Hepatitis B (HepB) and Haemophilus influenza type B vaccines.[260] By 2006 (figure 3), there had been substantial changes with the whole cell DTP, now replaced with the acellular pertussis containing DTaP, and with the oral polio vaccine (OPV), replaced with the injected inactivated polio vaccine (IPV). There was also the addition of varicella, pneumococcal conjugate (PCV), influenza, and Hepatitis A (HepA) vaccines.[261] Between the 1995 and 2006 schedules, a Rotavirus vaccine was recommended and then quickly withdrawn due to an association with intussusception.[262] In the 2013 immunization schedule (figure 4), the only dramatic change from the 2006 schedule for preschoolers was a new Rotavirus recommendation.[263]

The recommended immunization schedule has become substantially more complex and harder to follow for parents and for immunization providers. The United States has gone from five injections and four oral doses of vaccines in the first six years of life in 1983 to potentially thirty-three injections and three oral doses of vaccine in 2013 (if influenza is given by injection and no combinations are used); the various available combination vaccines further complicate this. These complexities and combination vaccines increase the possibility that this key component of well-child care, vaccines, will not be effectively delivered. Combination vaccines are helpful in reducing the number of injections that a child has to receive at any one visit. However, careful thought and planning has to go into the decisions regarding what vaccine combinations to stock and give to avoid confusion and either failing to provide needed doses of vaccine or overvaccinating children.

Immunization Delivery to Children

As part of the US Morbidity Study from 1928 to 1931, the first collection of utilization data for vaccines in common use was performed. The data collected were for smallpox, diphtheria, typhoid fever, and scarlet fever vaccines. This survey found that the most common immunization of preschool children was against diphtheria, reaching a peak of about 43 percent at nine years of age. Most children were not immunized until entry into school, at which point smallpox vaccination was the most prominent.

By sixteen years of age, 66 percent had received smallpox vaccination.²⁶⁴

The advent of polio vaccine in the 1950s marked the first attempt by the United States to estimate poliomyelitis vaccination coverage. After an initial attempt to estimate vaccination coverage using information provided by manufacturers-produced results that were difficult to interpret, the CDC requested that the Bureau of the Census add questions on poliomyelitis vaccination to the Current Population Survey.²⁶⁵ This survey became known as the US Immunization Survey (USIS), and with additional questions on new vaccines added from 1957 to 1985, household-reported vaccination histories were used to estimate national vaccination coverage rates.²⁶⁶

Immunization data has also been collected as part of the National Health Interview Survey (NHIS) from 1991 to the present.²⁶⁷ The annual National Immunization Survey (NIS) began in 1994 for children and in 2008 for teens. The NIS has advantages over previous surveys in that it validates household-reported receipt of vaccines through a provider survey, and it generates state-level estimates of immunization coverage.²⁶⁸ Specifically, the NIS estimates the immunization rate at two years of age gathered by surveying the parents of children eighteen to thirty-five months of age, followed by a survey of identified immunization providers to confirm immunization receipt by the children surveyed. The immunization estimates that follow in this chapter are based on the NIS for children.

Goals for Immunization Delivery

Every ten years, the Public Health Service sets goals for the next ten years. The current goals are published as part of HealthyPeople 2020. The immunization goals for preschool children are stated in two different ways.

- To examine routinely each of the recommended vaccines, and the goal is related to that specific vaccine. For instance, the goal (IID-7.5) for polio vaccine is that 90

percent of children nineteen to thirty-five months will have received three or more doses of polio vaccine.[269]
- To examine a specific set of vaccines and whether children have received those immunizations. This is usually referred to as vaccine series complete. For instance, goal IID-8 is that 80 percent of children nineteen to thirty-five months of age will have received the recommended doses of all of these vaccines: DTaP, polio, MMR, Hib, hepatitis B, varicella, and PCV.[270]

For most of the individual antigens, as for the polio vaccine above, the goal is receipt of the appropriate vaccines by 90 percent of children between nineteen and thirty-five months of age. The fourth column of table 1 lists the goal for the vaccine listed in the first column.

The individual HealthyPeople 2020 vaccine objectives are that 90 percent of children should receive four or more doses of DTP/DT/DTaP, three or more doses of polio, one or more doses of MMR, three or more doses of Hib, three or more doses of Hepatitis B, one or more doses of varicella, and four or more doses of pneumococcal conjugate vaccine. Hepatitis B series is recommended to be started at birth, and the objective for this vaccine is 85 percent receiving two or more immunizations. Hepatitis A immunization is recommended to be at least 85 percent, and at least 80 percent is recommended for the completed Rotavirus series (see table 1). The HealthyPeople 2020 objective for vaccine series is that 80 percent of children nineteen to thirty-five months of age receive the vaccines recommended prior to those months, which are 4:3:1:3:3:1:4 (four or more doses of DTaP/DT/DTP, three or more doses of poliovirus vaccine, one or more doses of any MMR vaccine, three or more Hib vaccine, three or more doses of HepB, one or more doses of varicella vaccine, and four or more doses of PCV). This series objective is a leading health indicator for preventive services in HealthyPeople 2020. The leading health indicators were selected to communicate high-priority health issues and actions that can be taken to address them.[271]

The United States is currently at historic vaccination levels. In figure 5, the measured immunization levels in preschool children from 1967 to 2011 are presented. On the Y axis is the percent of the population covered, with the X axis showing the year. The top heavy black line near the top of the graph is the ninetieth percentile coverage level and represents the HealthyPeople 2020 objective for individual vaccines, with the exception of Rotavirus vaccine, where the objective is 80 percent.[272] Each of the lines represents an individual vaccine, with the number of doses to be up-to-date in parentheses. The period from 1967 to 1985 was measured with the USIS, the National Health Interview Survey from 1991 to 1993, and the NIS from 1994 to present. Note that the years from 1986 to 1991, represented by dotted lines, are a period when there was no national measurement of immunization rates.

Table 1 presents the vaccination coverage among children nineteen to thirty-five months of age in 2011 in the United States for selected vaccines and vaccine series. Also shown are the states with the lowest coverage, the highest coverage, and what the HealthyPeople 2020 percent coverage (if available) is for that vaccine or vaccine series. The United States as a whole has reached the HealthyPeople 2020 objectives for many of the individual vaccines, including poliovirus, MMR, Hib, Hepatitis B, and varicella vaccines. The objectives have not been reached for DTaP, Hepatitis B birth dose, PCV, Hepatitis A, and the full series of Rotavirus vaccines. It is worth noting that for almost all of the individual vaccine objectives, there is a state that has met the objective. The exceptions are the Hepatitis B birth dose and Hepatitis A (which is both new and given in the second year of life). We are far from meeting the 4:3:1:3:3:1:4 series objective, though this may still be an effect of the Hib shortage from December 2007 to September 2009.[273] Table 1 also presents the same series but without Hib (4:3:1:3:0:1:4). Note that although the coverage is higher, it still does not meet the HealthyPeople 2020 series objective.

Table 1: Vaccination coverage levels among children 19–35 months, 2011[a]

Vaccine (Doses)	Lowest State	Highest State	US Coverage	Healthy People 2020 Objective[274]	Oklahoma
DTP/DT/DTaP (≥4)[b]	75	92	85	90	84[275]
Poliovirus (≥3)[c]	86	99	94	90	94[276]
MMR (≥1)[d]	86	97	92	90	94[277]
Hib (≥3)[e]	86	97	94	90	93[278]
Hepatitis B (≥3)[f]	82	97	91	90	93[279]
Hepatitis B Birth Dose[g]	23	83	67	85	71[280]
Varicella (≥1)[h]	84	94	91	90	91[281]
PCV (≥3)[i]	87	99	94	NA	93[282]
PCV (≥4)[j]	74	94	84	90	80[283]
Hepatitis A (≥2)[k]	29	69	52	85	63[284]
Rotavirus Full Series[l]	52	80	67	80	58[285]
4:3:1[m]	73	92	83	NA	84[286]
4:3:1:0:3:1:4[n]	62	84	74	NA	73[287]
4:3:1:3:3:1:4[o,p]	58	79	69	80	66[288]

Children in the Q1/2011-Q4/2011 National Immunization Survey were born from January 2008 through May 2010.

- 4 or more doses of any diphtheria and tetanus toxoids and pertussis vaccines, including diphtheria, tetanus toxoids, and any acellular pertussis vaccine (DTaP/DTP/DT)
- 3 or more doses of any poliovirus vaccine

Well-Child Care in Infancy

- 1 or more doses of measles-mumps-rubella vaccine
- 3 or more doses of *Haemophilus influenzae* type b (Hib) vaccine
- 3 or more doses of Hepatitis B vaccine
- 1 or more doses of Hepatitis B vaccine administered between birth and age 3 days
- 1 or more doses of varicella at or after child's first birthday, unadjusted for history of varicella illness
- 3 or more doses of pneumococcal conjugate vaccine (PCV)
- 4 or more doses of PCV
- 2 or more doses of Hepatitis A vaccine
- ≥2 or ≥3 doses of Rotavirus vaccine, depending on product type received (≥2 doses for Rotarix® [RVI] or ≥3 doses for RotaTeq® [RV5])
- 4 or more doses of DTaP, 3 or more doses of poliovirus vaccine, and 1 or more doses of any MMR vaccine
- 4:3:1 plus 3 or more doses of HepB vaccine, 1 or more doses of varicella vaccine, and 4 or more doses of PCV; Hib vaccine is excluded
- 4:3:1 plus 3 or more doses Hib vaccine, 3 or more doses of HepB, 1 or more doses of varicella vaccine, and 4 or more doses

Clinical Effectiveness

Diseases prevented by routine vaccination are at or near historic lows (table 2). For most vaccine-preventable diseases, the incidence of disease has decreased from 95 percent to 100 percent. The exception is pertussis, which is now at the highest level in fifty years, as seen in figure 2.[289] The last case of paralytic polio in the Western hemisphere occurred in 1991.[290] Smallpox was declared eradicated in 1980.[291] Endemic transmission of measles was found to have ceased in 2000,[292] and in 2003 rubella was declared eliminated from the United States.[293]

Table 2: Impact of vaccines in the United States[294]

Disease	Prevaccine Annual Morbidity	2010 Total	% Decrease
Smallpox	29,005	0	100
Diphtheria	21,053	0	100
Pertussis	200,752	27,550	86
Tetanus	580	26	96
Polio (paralytic)	16,316	0	100
Measles	503,217	63	>99.9
Mumps	162,344	2,612	98
Rubella	47,745	5	>99.9
Congenital rubella syndrome	152	0	100
Invasive *Haemophilus influenza* type b (<5 years)	20,000	246*	99
Hepatitis A	117,333	1,670	99
Acute hepatitis B	66,232	3,374	95
Invasive pneumococcal disease (<5 years)	16,069	2,186	86
Rotavirus (hospitalizations <5 years old)	62,500	2,500	96
Varicella	4,085,120	15,427	>99.6

* Serotype b or unknown serotype

More recently introduced vaccines have had a dramatic effect on morbidity. Examples of the effects seen include the following.

- Pneumococcal vaccine has resulted in reductions in pneumococcal meningitis, pneumonia, and frequent otitis media in children.[295]
- With the varicella vaccine, there has been a decline in hospitalizations.[296]
- Hepatitis A vaccination has resulted in fewer outpatient visits and hospitalizations.[297]

- Rotavirus vaccination has resulted in fewer hospitalizations and reduced diarrhea associated with reduced health-care utilization and expenditures.[298] In fact, with the introduction of Rotavirus vaccine, the epidemiology of the disease appears to have changed with the disappearance of the typical southwest to northeast spread of Rotavirus activity.[299] The 2010–2011 season was eight weeks shorter than the prevaccine baseline, and in 2011–2012, the national threshold for the start of the Rotavirus season was never achieved.[300]

The introduction of the measles vaccine and its effect on disease burden can serve as an illustrative case. In the pre-vaccine era, there were an estimated three to four million cases of measles annually (much of the birth cohort) with 500,000 cases and 500 deaths reported to the CDC. In 1963, measles vaccine was licensed in the United States, and the incidence of measles fell precipitously; by 1983 only 1,497 cases were reported. The inset in figure 6 shows a resurgence of measles cases in 1989–1991; over those years, there were 55,622 cases and 123 deaths reported. The major reason for this epidemic of measles was unvaccinated children. With the subsequent redoubling of immunization efforts spurred by this epidemic, the incidence of measles was substantially decreased, and as noted above, measles is no longer endemic in the United States.[301] In 2004, a record low number of 37 measles cases were reported, and in 2010, there were 63 cases of measles reported in the United States. Almost all cases were epidemiologically linked to an imported case.

In contrast, pertussis or whooping cough serves as something of a cautionary tale (see figure 7). Since 1982, even before the introduction of the acellular pertussis vaccine, the incidence of pertussis was climbing. With the introduction of the acellular pertussis vaccines as DTaP and then Tdap (for adolescents), there has been a dramatic increase in pertussis, with the incidence in 2010 being the highest in fifty years, though it is still much lower than in the epidemic years of the 1930s. This increase in pertussis is probably related to vaccines that are not as efficacious as the previous vaccines, PCR technology that improves detection of disease, and increased awareness of the disease by physicians.[302]

Economic Impact

The routine immunization of preschool children prevents disease and saves lives. Zhou et al. examined the economics of routine immunization of children six years and under in 2001.[303] Rodewald et al. updated this analysis for current research, and currently recommended vaccines can be seen in table 3. Overall, the routine immunization of these children has prevented almost 20 million cases of disease and 42,000 deaths from those diseases in each birth cohort. Accounting for the costs of vaccination, this represents a $6.7 billion direct and $7.5 billion societal cost savings. These figures can be subtracted to determine the net present value of the US program: $13.5 billion direct and $69 billion to society. The benefit to cost ratio is three to one (20.28/7.5) for direct costs and ten to one (76.4:7.5) costs to society for immunizing the 2009 birth cohort.

The Partnership for Prevention has used an explicit system to prioritize preventive services. This method uses both the clinical burden of disease as a measure of the particular health-service impact and the cost-effectiveness of the service as a measure of economic value.[304] They evaluated the clinical preventive services that were considered effective by the US Preventive Services Task Force and the Advisory Committee on Immunization Practices. Immunizations for children were among the three highest-ranking preventive services, achieving the highest rank for both reduced clinical burden of disease and cost-effectiveness.[305]

Well-Child Care in Infancy

Table 3: Lifetime economic impact of vaccinating the 2009 US birth cohort using the immunization schedule for children six years or younger, not including influenza vaccine[306]

Disease	Cases	Deaths	Direct Costs*	Societal Costs (Direct and Indirect)*
Diphtheria	275,028	27,503	3,654	39,296
Tetanus	169	25	12	45
Pertussis	2,950,836	1,062	4,450	7,024
Polio	67,463	800	2,898	7,259
Measles	3,835,825	3,106	3,763	8,863
Mumps	2,312,275	12	1,416	2,379
Rubella	1,981,066	15	187	721
Congenital rubella syndrome	632	70	133	257
Haemophilus influenza type b	19,606	741	1,810	3,756
Varicella	4,069,435	72	383	1,643
Hepatitis B	237,956	3,491	239	1,759
Hepatitis A	153,164	36	52	114
Pneumococcus-related diseases	2,323,952	5,056	965	2,696
Rotavirus	1,592,294	18	322	589
Total	19,819,701	42,007	20,284	76,401

* Costs are in millions of dollars.

William B. Pittard III, MD, PhD, MPH

Summary

The immunization of children prevents morbidity and mortality and is perhaps the most effective and cost-effective component of well-child care. The effect that the routine immunization program has had on the health of children is profound. Yet as the measles epidemic of 1989–1991 demonstrates, failure to vaccinate will result in the return of these vaccine-preventable diseases. As pertussis demonstrates, there will also be the need to develop better vaccines and to think creatively about how best to use them to fight disease.

Despite the challenges and failures as well as highlighting the successes of the effort to immunize children, the development and dissemination of vaccines is one of the greatest achievements of biomedical science and public health.[307]

Figure 1: Recommended schedule for active immunization of normal infants and children (United States, 1983)[308]

Vaccine ▼ / Age ►	2 mo	4 mo	6 mo	15 mo	18 mo	4-6 y	14-16 y
Diphtheria, Tetanus, Pertussis	DTP	DTP	DTP		DTP	DTP	Td
Oral Poliovirus vaccine	OPV	OPV			OPV	OPV	
Measles, Mumps, Rubella				MMR			

Well-Child Care in Infancy

Figure 2: Recommended childhood immunization schedule—United States, January 1995[309]

Vaccine	Birth	2 Months	4 Months	6 Months	12† Months	15 Months	18 Months	4-6 Years	11-12 Years	14-16 Years
Hepatitis B§	HB-1	HB-2		HB-3						
Diphtheria, Tetanus, Pertussis¶		DTP	DTP	DTP	DTP or DTaP at ≥15 months			DTP or DTaP	Td	
H. influenzae type b**		Hib	Hib	Hib	Hib					
Poliovirus		OPV	OPV	OPV				OPV		
Measles, Mumps, Rubella††					MMR			MMR or MMR		

Figure 3: Recommended childhood and adolescent immunization schedule—United States, January 2006[310]

Vaccine ▼ / Age ▶	Birth	1 month	2 months	4 months	6 months	12 months	15 months	18 months	24 months	4-6 years	11-12 years	13-14 years	15 years	16-18 years
Hepatitis B¹	HepB	HepB		HepB¹		HepB					HepB Series			
Diphtheria, Tetanus, Pertussis²			DTaP	DTaP	DTaP		DTaP			DTaP	Tdap	Tdap		
Haemophilus influenzae type b³			Hib	Hib	Hib³	Hib								
Inactivated Poliovirus			IPV	IPV		IPV				IPV				
Measles, Mumps, Rubella⁴						MMR				MMR	MMR			
Varicella⁵						Varicella					Varicella			
Meningococcal⁶									Vaccines within broken line are for selected populations MPSV4		MCV4	MCV4		MCV4
Pneumococcal⁷			PCV	PCV	PCV	PCV			PCV		PPV			
Influenza⁸						Influenza (yearly)				Influenza (yearly)				
Hepatitis A⁹						HepA series				HepA series				

Figure 4: Recommended immunization schedule for persons aged zero through eighteen years—United States, 2013[311]*

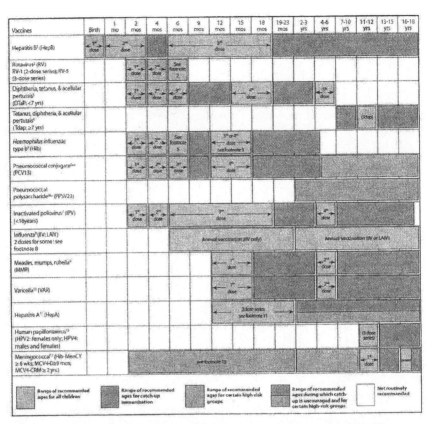

*The footnotes are an intergral part of the immunization schedule. They can be found at the CDC website at http://www.cdc.gov/vaccines/schedules/hcp/child-adolescent.html.

Figure 5: Vaccination coverage levels of preschool children in the United States from 1967 through June 2011[312]

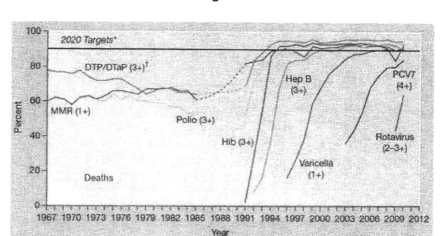

*HealthyPeople 2020 targets are 90 percent except for Rotavirus vaccine, which is 80 percent. The numbers in parentheses indicate the number of doses required to be considered up-to-date for the vaccine. For Rotavirus vaccine, the number of doses needed depends on the specific vaccine used.

†DTP(3+) is not a HealthyPeople 2010 objective. DTaP(4) is used to assess HealthyPeople 2010 objectives.

Note: During the years connected by dotted lines, there was no national coverage measurement system. Children in the USIS and National Health Interview Survey (NHIS) were 24–35 months old. Children in the National Immunization Survey (NIS) were 19–35 months old. Data sources: USIS (1967–1985); NHIS (1991–1993); NIS (1994–2010).

Figure 6: The effect of the introduction of measles vaccine in the US[313]

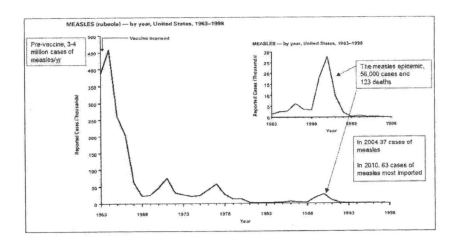

Figure 7: Pertussis incidence* by year—United States, 1980–2010[314]

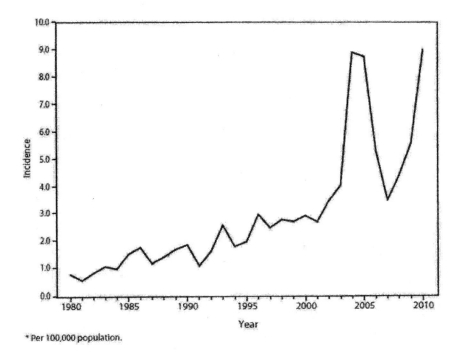

* Per 100,000 population.

CHAPTER 6

Well-Child Care in a Changing US Delivery System

Oscar Lovelace, MD
William B. Pittard III, MD, PhD, MPH

Introduction

Well-child care training for primary care providers (PCPs) has long relied on the core set of age-specific preventive-care guidelines recommended by the American Academy of Pediatrics (AAP).[315] These guidelines cover an array of topics regarding dietary intake, sleep position, and developmental assessment under the headings of parental anticipatory guidance, screening procedures, and immunizations. An additional component of well-child care is an age-based physical examination. As children grow, the time spent by PCPs teasing out critical nutritional and psychosocial issues during the well-child visit may have a far greater impact on a child's reaching his or her growth and developmental potential than is currently documented in the literature. For example, a well-child care priority today must be on addressing the national epidemic of childhood obesity.[316] Although PCPs are clearly aware of the AAP recommendations for the number and content of well-child visits, there are few published guidelines or recommendations regarding how to uniquely tailor the delivery of well-child care to the individual genetic, cultural, physical, and psychosocial needs of different children.[317]

This chapter addresses the government's role in well-child care, including access points, cost barriers, and the role of the Balanced Budget Act and Medicaid. It then discusses the private sector's role. Providers are faced with the challenge of prioritizing the perceived needs of parents and children to fit the limited time available for well-child visits. These needs include the more traditional preventive-care services, as well as newer issues such as obesity, depression, behavioral problems, and attention-deficit/hyperactivity disorder. This chapter discusses this provider concern, the governmental and economic forces that impact the delivery and content of well-child care today. Finally, the chapter discusses policy, opportunity, and the systemic changes these forces may require for well-child care in the near future.

The Government's Role in Well-Child Care

In America, state and federal government regulations have arguably played a greater role in determining what is expected in the provision of well-child care in recent years. In April 2012, the Center for Medicaid and Medicare Services (CMS) published an advisory on the initiation of G-codes for Medicare beneficiaries, which offered additional PCP reimbursement for the provision and documentation of screening and office-based counseling for obesity, depression, alcoholism, and cardiovascular disease.[318] This guideline followed an earlier policy providing reimbursement for tobacco-use screening and office-based smoking-cessation counseling.[319] These changes represent evidence-based policy implementation of the US Preventive Services Task Force recommendations for adults. In this case, Medicare is taking a lead role in transforming our health-care delivery system and acknowledging the critical importance of preventive and primary care. Well-child care has little to do with Medicare, but Medicaid policy makers could enact similar regulations to promote preventive and primary care utilization by children.

Changing the Emergency Department (ED) Access Point to Address Cost per Patient

In October 2007, US Comptroller General David Walker convincingly demonstrated in a report from the GAO (Government Accountability Office) entitled "Fiscal and Healthcare Challenges" that the demography and aging of the US population is not the critical issue facing our nation's health care.[320] The looming fiscal crisis is not the number of patients but the rising cost per patient. Understandably, beneficiary costs are far greater for adults in Medicare than for children more commonly enrolled in Medicaid. However, since the passage of the Affordable Care Act, and more recently the Supreme Court's recognition of its constitutionality, there will be a significant increase in Medicaid beneficiaries, and secondarily in services utilized.[321] This expansion should encourage policy changes within Medicaid, similar to the G-codes currently available to providers of Medicare services. Otherwise, the shortage of providers and the underuse of Medicaid preventive-care services by children will lead to further escalation of health-care costs.

Barrier to Well-Child Care Provision and Utilization

Several specific concerns of PCPs serve to limit the provision of well-child and preventive care to children.[322] These barriers include low reimbursement for preventive care and developmental screenings for children by providers and staff, inadequate provider training in screening procedures, and limited access to and communication with community, family, and child-support facilities. Last, an anticipated cost increase is the inevitable consequence of acute but not preventive care being provided to low-income individuals by the current universal health-care access point, the hospital emergency department (ED), rather than from a medical home.[323] Indeed, in 2010, the average hospital ED charge was $1,349.[324] In comparison, the average cost for an office-based physician visit was $199 (specialist and primary care). Although these values are skewed, the median cost for an ED and a physician office visit was $615 and $89, respectively.[325]

Quasi-Standardization of Well-Child Care

The paucity of empirical data documenting clinical effectiveness for much of the content of well-child care has been frequently noted.[326] Indeed, the AAP recommendations for both the number and content of well-child care were originally based solely on consensus expert opinion rather than investigation.

When Medicaid was established in 1965, the child-care focus was all but entirely confined to acute medical services.[327] Almost immediately, the need for a broader scope including preventive care was apparent. Although the information gap regarding well-child care clinical effectiveness was clearly recognized by the AAP in the early 1970s, this deficiency continued for more than three decades after the original recommendations were established.[328] Recognizing the need for preventive care, federal policy makers established a comprehensive well-child Medicaid benefit specifically for children in 1967 called Early and Periodic Screening, Diagnosis, and Treatment (EPSDT).[329]

The elements of EPSDT are reflected by its name.[330]

Early	Identifying problems early, starting at birth
Periodic	Checking children's health at periodic, age-appropriate intervals
Screening	Performing physical, mental, developmental, dental, hearing, vision, and other screening procedures to detect potential problems
Diagnosis	When risk is identified, conducting appropriate follow-up diagnostic tests
Treatment	Treating identified problems

This benefit addresses the unique physical, mental, and developmental preventive-care needs of low-income children. Since creation, the purpose of EPSDT, as stated in the federal rule, has been "to discover, as early as possible, the ills that handicap our children" and to provide "continuing follow-up and treatment so that handicaps do not go neglected."[331] Federal law mandates through a variety of statutes, regulations, and guidelines that Medicaid must include this very comprehensive set of preventive-care services for children, different from adult benefits.[332]

The Balanced Budget Act of 1997 and the State Child Health-Insurance Programs

Until the mid-1980s, Medicaid enrollment by children was almost entirely composed of those living in families eligible for Aid to Families with Dependent Children (AFDC). However, beginning in 1984, Congress enacted legislation on a yearly basis, expanding Medicaid eligibility to children far beyond those simply in AFDC families.[333] Then, following the creation of the State Children's Health Insurance Program (SCHIP) via the Balanced Budget Act of 1997, many more children became eligible for Medicaid.[334] Nevertheless, because Medicaid eligibility was closely tied to AFDC during its first three decades of existence, it inappropriately became a welfare program in the minds of many, and today Medicaid enrollment carries a social stigma.[335]

Medicaid Eligibility

Until 1996, Medicaid was administered with Aid to Families with Dependent Children (AFDC) and the Supplemental Security Income (SSI) program, both government cash-assistance agencies for low-income individuals. Although eligibility requirements for SSI were set by federal law, AFDC eligibility was set by each individual state even though it was a federal grant-in-aid program. Perhaps of greater concern to many was the fact that because AFDC eligibility established most children's eligibility for Medicaid, states trying to remove the working poor from their AFDC role by lowering AFDC eligibility denied Medicaid and its preventive-care benefit to many low-income children.[336] This limitation for working poor families was particularly egregious because more than half of all low-income children lived in families with at least one working member. Because minimum wage earners are infrequently offered health insurance as a fringe benefit, more than half of the uninsured Americans were either members of or dependents in working poor families.[337] After the 1996 Personal Responsibility and Work Opportunity Reconciliation Act (PRWORA) delinked eligibility for Medicaid from eligibility for cash-assistance programs, many children who were eligible for Medicaid were not enrolled.[338]

Because the incidence of poverty among children increased in 1996 and was associated with a reduction in Medicaid enrollment, concern existed that states may be removing children from Medicaid whose families were no longer enrolled in public assistance despite their continued eligibility for Medicaid.[339] Prior to 1996, families with dependent children receiving cash assistance via AFDC were automatically eligible for Medicaid. The PRWORA did away with AFDC and replaced it with the Temporary Assistance for Needy Families (TANF) program. Eligibility for TANF is available only for a five-year period, is based on more strict resource requirements, and includes mandatory work requirements.

The Federal Balanced Budget Act of 1997, which created the State *Children's* Health Insurance Programs (SCHIPs), also allowed states to further expand their Medicaid enrollment with its EPSDT benefit or to establish the new SCHIP program with or without the EPSDT benefit.[340] Unlike Medicaid, which is a state- and federal-funded individual entitlement program, the SCHIP is block grant funded and is an entitlement to the individual states rather than to the enrolled children.[341] As a result, even prior to the planned Medicaid expansion in 2013, 36 percent of US children were enrolled in Medicaid.[342]

The Deficit Reduction Act of 2005 (DRA, enacted February 2006) gave states more options to modify the approach to delivery of services to children enrolled in Medicaid.[343] These Medicaid service delivery changes had direct impact on the EPSDT benefit. For example, the DRA allows states to restructure their approach to Medicaid benefits without a federal waiver using the state plan amendment process. The DRA also included a more specific definition of case management and placed limits on use of targeted and administrative case management, which allows variation in the delivery of Medicaid services for infants, children, and adolescents. With this legislation, many states created state-run medical home programs or clinic systems for Medicaid patients, or in special circumstances contracted with out-of-state enrollment entities and managed-care organizations to enroll patients and manage the Medicaid benefits for children.

Impact of Increased Medicaid Eligibility on Health-Care Delivery

It is unlikely that private payers will drive the changes needed to implement best-practice well-child care in our nation's somewhat fractured health-care delivery system. Although one-third of all US children are currently Medicaid eligible, in poorer states well over half of all children below age six years are eligible. With the planned expansion of Medicaid eligibility in 2013, there is concern by some about having an adequate supply of PCPs (including physicians, physician assistants, and nurse practitioners) in the near future to deliver the required services.[344]

With these concerns, it is understandable that state and federal government agencies are trying to redefine the service content of well-child care as a cost-saving mechanism. This approach increases the need for focused investigation assessing the clinical effectiveness of well-child preventive-care services. An example of this is that states have shown significant cost savings and quality of care improvement with primary care Medical Home Programs for both medically fragile and less high-risk children.[345] Clearly, the forces of politics have greatly influenced the direction individual states have taken in the management and implementation of Medicaid reform efforts. This program is jointly funded by state and federal matching funds, and eligibility is variably set by each individual state based on family income levels. This distinguishes Medicaid from Medicare, which is entirely federally funded. A federal policy change rapidly results in systemic change for all Medicare beneficiaries throughout the nation, whereas states are allowed much greater managerial control with Medicaid. Some states have chosen to outsource their enrollment and payment for services to the managed-care insurance industry, and others have continued to use public service employees to perform these tasks.

William B. Pittard III, MD, PhD, MPH

The Private-Sector Role in Well-Child Care

Unlike salaried practitioners in hospitals or various managed-care organizations, PCPs in the community setting, as a group, are often referred to as private-sector physicians. For both privately and Medicaid insured children, data demonstrating improvement in the cost and quality of care with enrollment in primary care patient-centered medical homes (PCMH) is impressive and is thought to reflect the benefits of continuity of care in a familiar setting with well-known and trusted caregivers.[346] With these observations, physicians in private practice are being encouraged to become credentialed as PCMH practitioners. However, few payers (private or governmental) have developed a reimbursement model to entice PCPs to incur the added expense of the credentialing process and the systemic changes in protocol and personnel required to effect this change.

Currently, there is another and possibly more dramatic change in our nation's health-care delivery taking place, with potential to adversely influence well-child care. An increasing number of PCPs are being employed by hospitals (hospitalists), and fewer are in private practice.[347] This phenomenon could have a direct impact on the implementation of new policy directives. Hospitalists may be less focused on new initiatives, choosing instead to let hospital administrators sort through novel coding and documentation requirements. On the other hand, hospital administrators have been less engaged in the nuances of primary care billing such as tracking down small co-pays, and they could be less interested in new, small, additional reimbursements or incentive payments offered for the provision of primary care preventive services.

Prioritizing the Recommended Well-Child Care Topics

Despite the many challenges, PCPs are and will continue to be depended upon for the delivery of preventive and well-child care. Pediatricians, family physicians, and nurse practitioners, via the anticipatory guidance portion of well-child care, must educate parents regarding cost-efficient treatment for childhood chronic illness and appropriate use of primary care services, including hospital EDs and PCP office visits.

There are several issues to consider when individualizing well-child care provision in the office setting. A provider's assessment of maternal-infant bonding and parenting skills represents the foundation for well-child care. If there is concern about an infant or child being in a dangerous or neglectful home situation, it is important to know how to engage community support systems such as child protective services. Fortunately, many high-risk home environments are identified during prenatal care and result in social service intervention prior to delivery.[348]

For the initial office visit postdelivery, it is imperative that the PCP review the hospital discharge summary to be aware of concerns identified and dealt with during the prenatal and immediate newborn period. Review of the prenatal course and neonatal hospitalization may facilitate a more focused postnatal examination, facilitate appropriate referrals, and enhance recognition of needed support. Pertinent information such as prenatal exposure to hepatitis B infection, need for neonatal resuscitation at delivery, or unique clinical findings in the newborn nursery, such as hip instability, may be described in the newborn hospital discharge summary. The presence or absence of the PCP during the neonatal hospitalization may indicate need for a closer assessment of medical or social issues. In situations where a hospitalist is discharging an infant or child to the community, it is mandatory that a discharge summary reach the child's PCP on the day of discharge, and significant issues should be communicated by phone.

A detailed history of the transition from hospital to home taken from the parent (including feeding, stooling and voiding, and sleep patterns, as well as medication compliance) and assessment of all parental concerns should guide the PCP in the initial infant well-child visit. A thorough understanding of the home environment obtained during well-child visits allows the PCP to effectively guide the trajectory of a child's life. Early brain and cognitive developmental investigation has highlighted the importance of daily routine in promoting optimal personal and social child development[349]. Although intuitively one might assume that a stay-at-home parent uniquely facilitates adequate and healthy psychosocial child development and eventually school readiness, essentially all parents need access to social support systems and child-rearing counseling available via their child's PCP as a portion of well-child care. Working parents often need help finding affordable, quality child care, because many child care centers fail to meet minimal standards. However, the developmental outcomes of children in approved daycare centers are impressive.[350]

After obtaining pertinent information from the parent or caregiver and considering the child's individual needs, PCPs then must conduct a thorough physical examination to provide comprehensive well-child care. For example, the early detection of an asymmetric red reflex and appropriate referral can preserve a child's vision for life. Accurate measurement of height and weight are as essential in well-child care as the more traditional measurements of blood pressure, pulse, and respiration. The PCP community has become disciplined in obtaining height and weight as the patients age. However, an accurate height and weight does not address America's fastest-growing epidemic—obesity. Height and weight not only need to be plotted to assess growth adequacy but the two measures together should be used to calculate body mass index (BMI) related to patient's age. Only with BMI can obesity be accurately assessed.[351]

Obese mothers are more likely to produce macrosomic infants and children,[352] and therefore the problem of energy imbalance and obesity in children with its adverse health outcomes begins during the prenatal period.[353] The increased incidence of obesity or abnormally high BMI translates into an alarming health disadvantage for many children and adolescents in the United States compared to those with a normal BMI. Indeed, obesity will affect nearly every aspect of a child's future, including infant mortality, low birth weight, injuries, homicide, illicit drug use, high-risk sex, depression, high rates of childhood illness, high rates of child poverty, lower educational achievement, and lower social mobility.[354] This has major implications not only for public health but also for economic and national security.[355] Indeed, the greater US investment in enhancing health-care delivery to the elderly (i.e., the G-codes) than to the young may, with the graying of America, actually serve to create an even larger future erosion of political power for the young.

Policy and Opportunities to Improve Well-Child Care

Several programs and opportunities are available to improve the provision of preventive care to children.

1) Referrals

For children in low-income or otherwise disadvantaged homes, referrals to available community support programs such as parenting classes, health department resources, and Head Start are of great value. The past history of dialogue between the county health department, social services, and the medical care provider has been tenuous at best in many communities, with great potential for improvement.

2) Increased Connectivity

In this regard, the advent of electronic medical records offers a real opportunity for increased connectivity between office and community resources. Interconnectedness is a central goal of the Health Information Exchange, which is part of the new Affordable Care Act. Early interaction can be pivotal in initiating community resource support for poor social conditions, which often precipitate a series of adverse events in the life of a child.[356]

Distinct, well-reimbursed transition of care codes were implemented in 2013 for Medicare beneficiaries, but most private payers and Medicaid have been slow to adopt or incentivize this care or early, postdischarge follow-up care for children. In order for a PCP to receive the transition of care reimbursement from Medicare, the provider must have telephone or electronic contact with the patient within two business days of discharge, and the provider must see the patient in the primary care outpatient setting within two weeks of discharge. This approach is particularly beneficial for the complicated newborn but also for most hospitalized children in need of chronic disease management such as asthma.

3) Consider a Universal Care Policy for Children

On an international perspective, though health care in America is the most expensive in the world, it has far from the most desirable patient-health outcomes. As noted in a recent edition of US Health in International Perspective, US children are more likely to die prior to age five when compared to other developed countries.[357] The only demographic in America to experience a longer comparative lifespan than in other countries are adults over age seventy-five, although US citizens actually rank twenty-seventh internationally in longevity. This may again reflect the lack of balance in our health-care delivery system, because those over age sixty-five have Medicare and access to a universal insurance system. There are other important outcome differences for society with our American health-care system. US children are more likely to live in poverty and be exposed to higher rates of income inequality than those in most developed counties. Perhaps even more alarming is the fact that despite the US average per capita health-care spending being twice as high annually as the second-most expensive health-care system in the entire world, the United States, internationally, ranks twenty-fifth in infant mortality and has greater rates of unintentional injuries, homicides, teen pregnancy, STDs, HIV/AIDs, illicit drug use, obesity, diabetes, heart disease, chronic lung disease, and disability than developed countries with lower health-care expenditure.[358]

This study identifies the need for health-care reform, but solutions are less apparent. Perhaps some form of universal primary care for all children should be considered. Today, every nation in the world (developed and underdeveloped), except America, provides universal primary care to all of its citizens, and at least twenty-five nations spend less per capita on health care and have lower rates of infant mortality and greater life expectancy than Americans.

Well-Child Care in Infancy

4) Actions to Benefit Staff and Physician from Increased Demand

With the planned expansion of Medicaid in 2013 to include nearly half of all children in the United States and the variation in eligibility requirements in state Medicaid programs, delivering the needed preventive-care services for infants and children may become challenging. Studies have shown improved outcomes with well-child care and its preventive services when there is collaboration between government and community agencies and providers.[359] Specific actions that have been shown to be beneficial include physician and office staff education, aligning reimbursement incentives, decreasing service redundancy, and use of community resources to facilitate delivery of preventive care and support services.[360]

5) Continued Investigation

Although there has only recently been patient-oriented evidence presented in the medical literature regarding well-child care clinical effectiveness other than for immunizations, and little or none regarding the most effective method of delivery of preventive services to infants and children, this information gap indicates the presence of fertile ground for future investigation. For example, recent studies have found that electronic medical records use improves developmental screening rates, risk assessment, and age-appropriate counseling via structured data entry, clinical information tools, access to longitudinal patient data, and improved interfaces with laboratory results.[361] Electronic recall or auto-dialer systems, as well as letters or postcards, have been used to improve immunization rates. Health-maintenance reminder features found on many EHRs alert PCPs about necessary or delinquent services, which allows more comprehensive delivery of preventive and chronic disease management services, both of which occur during well-child care.[362]

All said, the most significant challenge has previously been noted as far back as biblical times: "the harvest is plentiful but the workers are few" (Luke 10:2).

CHAPTER 7

Well-Child Care: A Prudent Investment for the Future

William B. Pittard III, MD, PhD, MPH

Introduction

Well-child care is designed to improve the health status of children, and the American Academy of Pediatrics (AAP) recommends a widely accepted national standard for the content of this preventive care.[363] The Medicaid well-child benefit is called Early and Periodic Screening, Diagnosis, and Treatment (EPSDT). Six EPSDT visits are recommended by the AAP in the first year of life, three in the second, two in the third, and one annually thereafter through age twenty. The content of these visits includes all AAP-recommended, age-based preventive-care services. In the preschool years, these services include a physical examination, immunizations, anticipatory guidance for parents or caregivers, and screening procedures for early detection of disease and for vision, hearing, cognitive, and dental disorders.[364]

The focus of EPSDT is preventive care, and there are three primary components.[365] The first is immunizations that provide primary preventive care and have been repeatedly shown to be effective in reducing infectious disease morbidity.[366] The second component is screening procedures for early detection of physical and developmental problems. With early detection, appropriate therapy can be initiated sooner with fewer complications, reduced cost, and improved outcomes. A third concentration of well-child care is parental anticipatory guidance, which is often delivered in a "medical home" setting and includes health education and counseling to support and reassure families.[367]

Although well-child care provides comprehensive preventive-care coverage, utilization of EPSDT and well-child services by both low-income and more affluent children has been inadequate.[368]

Because empirical investigation was unavailable to the AAP when recommendations for well-child care were originally established, they were based on consensus expert opinion.[369] Confirmation of clinical effectiveness for these recommendations other than for immunizations and some screening procedures remained unavailable for more than three decades. Only in the last six years have empirical findings indicating effectiveness for the parental anticipatory guidance component of well-child care been available.[370]

Due to the long delay in confirming well-child care effectiveness, private- and public-insurance administrators have historically been uncertain whether implementing methods to correct the underuse of well-child care are worth the added cost.[371] Private-insurance policies rarely offer coverage for preventive services such as well-child care, and when offered they almost inevitably require a co-payment limiting utilization.[372] In contrast, the EPSDT benefit, which is government funded, has been less frequently used by low-income children than well-child care by children privately insured.[373] Of equal inconsistency is the finding that despite lack of utilization by children and with little empiric confirmation of effectiveness, it has been widely accepted by providers and many parents that this preventive care improves the health status of children.[374] This broad acceptance has been reflected by the argument offered in past publications that the absence of empirical confirmation of well-child care effectiveness should not be construed as evidence of ineffectiveness.[375]

As an overview, this chapter first offers a review of Medicaid, its mission, financial infrastructure, and large expansion in eligible beneficiaries and cost. A discussion of managed care, used as a method to control Medicaid cost, is provided. This discussion is followed with a summary of earlier and more recent findings regarding well-child care clinical effectiveness assessed using the holistic approach of comparing the health status of children that receive all components of the recommended number of well-child visits with the outcomes for those that receive fewer visits.[376] Health-service utilization by children enrolled in health-care models using different types of financing and delivery of medical care and health-status outcome differences by children through the preschool years are also noted.[377] Lastly, the cost-effectiveness of short- and longer-term health-status outcomes associated with receipt of the recommended well-child care by preschool children is discussed.[378]

Historical Review of Medicaid

Medicaid was established in 1965 as a federal-state entitlement program to finance health care for certain categories of low-income individuals.[379] The primary goal for Medicaid since its inception has been to provide the uninsured with access to routine primary care. Striking accelerations in Medicaid expenditure occurred during the 1980s, and expenses became almost hyperinflationary in the 1990s. These increases were secondary to both expanded eligibility and the expensive technology of medical care.[380] As a means of cost containment and improvement in budget predictability, throughout the 1980s and 1990s managed-care health-care models were progressively introduced into state Medicaid systems nationwide to replace the more traditional fee-for-service (FFS) model. Many different managed-care models were used with unique structural designs, but all shared the common goals of controlling cost and improving the quality of care. With this change to managed care came striking alterations in health-care delivery for beneficiaries both children and adults.

The federal financial participation (FFP), or share of Medicaid expenditures paid, is based on the average per capita income for each state. The minimum federal rate is 50 percent (in thirteen states), and the maximum rate is 80 percent (in one state), with a national average of 57 percent. Medicaid is run by federal, state, and local governments, and most states administer Medicaid through their county welfare agencies. At the federal level, the Centers for Medicare and Medicaid Services (CMS), previously known as the Health Care Financing Administration (HCFA) of the Department of Health and Human Services (DHHS), is the primary regulatory agency.[381] Medicaid has today become

America's dominant health-care financing mechanism for low-income children and has served to more nearly equalize access to primary health care between low-income and higher-income children.[382]

Shortly after Medicaid's initiation, it was apparent that in order to be more effective for children, Medicaid needed to have its coverage expanded from simply acute medical care to include preventive care as well. In 1967, two years after Medicaid's establishment, the Early and Periodic Screening, Diagnosis, and Treatment (EPSDT) benefit was added to Medicaid.[383] Data from the 1980s indicate that Medicaid coverage specifically increased access to primary health-care services for poor, otherwise uninsured children.[384] Unfortunately, data have also shown that simply providing low-income children with insurance coverage (access to care) does not guarantee utilization of health-care services, and certainly not to the same extent as more affluent children.[385] Lack of utilization of available Medicaid services by low-income children is in part because outreach education to parents regarding service availability and service need by children has been limited.[386] Further, many eligible children are not enrolled in Medicaid. In these areas, by some estimates, Medicaid has underserved more than one-third of low-income children in America.[387]

Changes in Medicaid Eligibility

Clearly, simply being poor does not automatically make an individual eligible for Medicaid. The five categories of eligible persons include families with dependent children, children under the age of twenty-one, pregnant women, older adults, and blind or disabled persons. The eligibility requirements for individuals in these specified categories are set by each state and therefore vary.

Until the mid-1980s, Medicaid enrollment by children was limited almost entirely to those living in families that qualified for Aid to Families with Dependent Children (AFDC). Beginning in 1984 and continuing until 1990, Congress enacted legislation on a yearly basis expanding Medicaid eligibility to many more children than simply those in AFDC families. Due to these expansions in eligibility, states were required to enroll children under age six in families with incomes up to 133 percent of poverty, and all children in families with incomes below the poverty level.[388] In addition, a number of states used waivers in the early 1980s to mid-1990s to further increase Medicaid coverage for parents and children.[389] Then, following the creation of the State Children's Health Insurance Program (SCHIP) via the Balanced Budget Act of 1997, even more children were eligible for Medicaid.[390]

Medicaid Managed Care to Control Cost

In the 1980s, Medicaid spending grew at an average annual rate of 5.9 percent, but it increased to an average of 9.8 percent in the 1990s. During 1993–1997, the number of Medicaid-eligible individuals increased from 28 to 41 million, with greater than 70 percent of the total being parents and their children.[391] The total Medicaid spending in 1980 was less than $25 billion, whereas in 1997 the total spending was greater than $159 billion. More interesting is the fact that in 1997, though 75 percent of the Medicaid-insured population was children and adults with dependent children, their cost was less than 30 percent of the total Medicaid expenditure. Thus 70 percent of all Medicaid expenditure was and is for the care of blind, aged, and disabled enrollees.[392]

An additional force that increased Medicaid cost and secondarily drove the initiation of cost-saving methodologies was an effort to infuse the principles of a market-driven economy into health care within the context of publicly funded care.[393] Because these two concepts are diametrically opposed, state Medicaid personnel found themselves torn between trying to provide equitable access to necessary health-care services and controlling spending. These competing goals are especially difficult to reach for high-risk populations such as the Medicaid-insured, due to the complexity of and costs associated with their health-care needs. A clear public health goal is to correct the underuse of needed services and to simultaneously control cost. Though these goals provide incentive for innovative thought, they are not consistent with a market-driven economy. There is no current consensus on the best approach to meet the needs of Medicaid recipients or the approaches that hold the most promise to reach the dual goal of providing equitable access to medical care and controlling cost.

With these rising Medicaid costs and in conjunction with the apparent success of managed care in containing private health-care expenditure, several states followed a proposal presented in the Omnibus Budget Reconciliation Act of 1981. This federal legislation encouraged states to develop new initiatives to curb costs using the Medicaid program waiver process. Using program waivers, states introduced different prepaid or managed-care case management plans into their Medicaid reform efforts.[394] Managed care, unlike fee-for-service (FFS), is more than simply a means of provider reimbursement for health-care services rendered. In fact, managed care is an arrangement that integrates both the financing and delivery of health-care services by a single organization for a defined population.[395]

What Is Managed Care?

Managed-care health plans fall along a continuum, reflecting several different infrastructural designs.[396] At one end of this continuum is managed indemnity or plans, which use precertification and maximum fee allowances to control provider utilization of services and co-payments, deductibles, and coinsurance to control patient service utilization. These forms of managed care are characteristic of most Blue Cross/Blue Shield programs today.

At the other end of the continuum are group and staff closed-panel health maintenance organizations (HMOs). Staff HMO physicians are employed by the HMO to care for enrollees, whereas group HMOs contract with a multispecialty group of physicians to provide care for enrollees, and these physicians are actually employed by the group, not by the HMO (e.g., Kaiser Permanente). The term "closed panel" simply means that PCPs who are not employed by the HMO (staff) or who are not part of the group contracted by the HMO cannot be reimbursed for providing services to an HMO beneficiary.

As one goes from left to right on this continuum, more restriction is applied by the managed-care models to control cost and service use. Therefore, there is no one single definition of the term "managed care," and managed-care models are not all alike. Specifically, managed-care models differ in terms of the degree of control they exert over patient and physician utilization of services or in their amount of integration between financing and delivery of care.

Does Managed Care Improve Medicaid Quality of Care and Limit Costs?

The fundamental question for Medicaid was and continues to be, is managed care more cost-effective than regular fee-for-service? Although low-income children and families represent approximately 70 percent of the Medicaid population nationally, they account for only approximately 30 percent of the annual cost. At the same time, the disabled and elderly represent approximately 25 percent of the Medicaid population but account for approximately 70 percent of the annual costs—that is, the so-called 70/30 rule.[397] This relationship partially explains why managed care has been less successful in controlling Medicaid expenditure than anticipated by some.

Originally, Medicaid managed care was projected to save 5–10 percent in annual costs based on reports in some private managed-care settings. This was to occur by (1) encouraging beneficiaries to obtain care from a single provider (a medical home) rather than from a nonprimary care provider source, (2) the promotion of routine preventive as well as medical care, (3) regulating the use of specialists, and (4) bargaining for lower rates with providers in return for a guaranteed patient load.[398]

There are at least three reasons why Medicaid managed care was unlikely to reach these original cost-saving projections.

- First, Medicaid programs primarily cover women and children—that is, about 70 percent of the Medicaid population accounts for approximately 25 percent of total Medicaid spending. Therefore, when the expected rate

Well-Child Care in Infancy

of 5–10 percent savings from Medicaid managed care is applied to this 25 percent of Medicaid expenditure, the overall Medicaid savings could only represent an approximate 1–2 percent total spending reduction.
- Second, Medicaid has traditionally paid providers a low reimbursement. Therefore, there is less room to negotiate discounted costs for a guaranteed patient load compared to commercial providers.
- Third, the Medicaid population needs more extensive outreach education and care-coordination efforts than the general public. Such services require increased expenditure, and thus it is really not surprising that managed care in a Medicaid population has failed to meet the expectations of some in limiting Medicaid costs.

Cost containment may also occur with improvement in quality of care as more healthy beneficiaries may require fewer healthcare services. If unnecessary and inappropriate service utilization is limited, the quality of care is enhanced, and the cost is reduced. On the other hand, if underuse of needed services is corrected, the quality of care is enhanced, but the cost is likely to be increased.[399] Therefore, with expansion in the number of eligible Medicaid beneficiaries from 1984 to 1990, many individuals who had previously been underusing needed health-care services were encouraged to more appropriately use these services with cost expansion rather than containment.

Medicaid-insured children have specifically been noted to use more emergency department (ED) visits than privately insured children for diagnoses routinely treated in a primary care provider (PCP) office or for nonurgent ambulatory care sensitive conditions (ACSCs).[400] This increased utilization of ACSC ED services by Medicaid children has been associated with receiving fewer than the recommended number of EPSDT visits in infancy.[401] Consistent with these observations, healthcare costs for Medicaid-enrolled children have been found to be greater in the preschool years than for privately insured children of the same age.[402]

William B. Pittard III, MD, PhD, MPH

Summary of Findings for Effectiveness

There have been both strengths and weaknesses noted with Medicaid managed care. The strengths include (1) slowing of the health expenditures (at least in the early 1990s), (2) lowering of hospital admission rates, (3) shortening the length of hospital stays, and (4) reducing the use of expensive procedures and tests.[403] The fourth strength has been associated with mixed outcome results, somewhat lower consumer satisfaction with services, and higher satisfaction with costs.[404] Also, at least an attempt has been made to eliminate waste and redundancy in the system.[405]

The primary weakness of managed care has been the simultaneous reduction in the power of physicians and hospitals to protect their professional and economic interests and to act independently in the interests of their patients.[406]

Because different mandatory managed-care models have become the dominant forms of health-care delivery for the Medicaid population, it is important to have a clear understanding of how different models of managed care affect beneficiaries. Comparisons of outcomes associated with FFS and managed care have often failed to address the fact that managed-care models are not all alike, and neither are all Medicaid populations. Therefore the outcomes of different managed-care models compare differently with the FFS model in different settings. This leads to difficulty in projecting the affect or efficacy of managed care in different communities, and this inability complicates policy planning and implementation. All too often the outcomes anticipated with managed-care models have erroneously been expected to occur with all forms of managed care in all Medicaid populations in an attempt to provide an expedient solution to rising health-care costs.

Well-Child Care Clinical Effectiveness

Early studies of well-child care effectiveness in improving the health status of children, published 1975–1990, used several different subpopulations of children and study designs and had very different findings, ranging from limited effectiveness to being unquestionably efficacious.[407] Though the global objective for well-child care is to improve the health status of children, confirming clinical effectiveness for individual components of this preventive-care system via empirical investigation has proven difficult for several reasons.

1) Clinical effectiveness of immunizations is confirmed differently than other components of well-child care.
2) The health status of children is more strongly influenced by social and economic factors than by medical care.
3) Few early studies of effectiveness used large enough sample sizes.
4) Because well-child care is broadly accepted as beneficial, randomized studies of clinical effectiveness are considered unethical.

Evidence for the effectiveness of immunizations is clearly established using randomized clinical trials as required for Federal Drug Administration licensing prior to being incorporated into the well-child care regimen.[408] In contrast, the effectiveness of other components of well-child care has not been as clearly demonstrated due to difficulties with experimental design.

The health status of children is driven by multiple factors and in general is more strongly influenced by social and economic factors than by medical or well-child care.[409] Specific contributing factors include family size, family income, urban or rural residence, and race and ethnicity.[410] Thus, studies to reliably detect the effect of well-child care, and certainly of individual components of this preventive care, require very large sample sizes.

Few early studies of well-child care effectiveness used large numbers of children. Further, because well-child care is widely accepted as beneficial to the health status of children by many parents and most providers, it is considered unethical to randomize children into study groups to receive and not to receive this preventive care, or to randomize them to receive certain but not all components of recommended well-child care. Therefore nonrandomized, quasi-experimental observational studies must be used, which allows documentation of significant associations but not the determination of causality per se.[411] These experimental design problems dictate a holistic evaluation of outcomes (effectiveness) observed among children that receive and do not receive the recommended number of well-child visits. To assess the effectiveness of individual well-child care components, one must simultaneously consider the specific objectives of each component part and the outcomes observed among children with and without the recommended well-child care. For example, immunizations are designed to limit infectious disease morbidity via primary preventive care, and anticipatory guidance is designed to provide parental health education to enhance optimal parenting behaviors such as getting children to effective health-care services, providing optimal nutrition, promoting exercise, and encouraging appropriate social and cognitive development to facilitate improved general health and school readiness.

Findings prior to 2000 assessing effectiveness of well-child care in promoting improved health status for children can be placed in three broad categories.[412]

- The first early findings category is that well-child care has little effect on childhood mortality. With the small sample sizes used and the relatively small number of actual deaths among children, the reliability of this finding is uncertain. Nevertheless, with reference to morbidity, two exemplary studies that assessed health status outcomes for children receiving different numbers of EPSDT visits are described. The first compared infants with six visits in the first year of life with those having only three visits.[413] The study found little difference in process-of-care measures, such as maternal satisfaction with care; it did not address objective measures of child health status such as the number of sick-child primary care provider (PCP) visits, the number of emergency department (ED) visits, or how well-child care specifically affected the health status of children. The second investigation compared the outcomes of children averaging 7.6 visits in the first two years of life with those

averaging 4.8 visits.[414] This study did not compare the outcomes for children receiving the AAP-recommended number of EPSDT visits with those receiving fewer visits, and it found no meaningful differences in health outcomes.
- The second category of early findings regarding well-child care effectiveness is that well-child care services may reduce the frequency of hospitalization. For example, it was reported that the general hospital admission rate (medical and surgical combined) for children cared for in a Rochester neighborhood clinic was 33 out of 1,000, versus 67 out of 1,000 for children in the same neighborhood not cared for in the clinic.[415] No information is provided regarding the well-child care received by either group, and only broad categorizations of admission diagnoses are provided. Thus, the understanding provided by this assessment regarding the clinical effectiveness of well-child care services, and more specifically by the individual components of well-child care in changing the rates of hospitalization or in improving the health status of children, is limited.
- The third category of early findings regarding well-child care effectiveness is that this preventive care had little effect on the developmental and social functioning of children.[416] Specific limitations of these studies included lack of generalizability or internal validity. Many of these studies have not been confirmed by more recent investigation using larger sample sizes.[417]

In summary, the literature prior to 2000 regarding the clinical effectiveness of well-child care was more noteworthy for its lack of reliable information than for the understanding it provided to stakeholders such as health-care providers, parents, children, and private-insurance or Medicaid policy makers. Specifically, no evidence was provided indicating that well-child care (other than immunization) influenced the morbidity or health status of children, or that it altered the development of social competence by children. The sample sizes used in these studies were too small, and the follow-up time was too short to draw valid conclusions regarding well-child care effectiveness. Few investigators assessed the impact duration of the well-child care effects they evaluated.

For many of these same reasons, expert opinion and good intentions were all that were available to the AAP to guide their initial recommendations for well-child care rather than scientific data.[418] The AAP well-child care recommendations and their utilization by preschool children were clearly driven for many years by parental and provider positive expectations rather than empiric evidence of effectiveness.

Recent Findings Regarding Well-Child Care Clinical and Cost-Effectiveness

After a prolonged delay in the generation of data indicating well-child care clinical effectiveness, findings since 2007 have offered a long-awaited response to this information gap. Using a collective or holistic approach, observational studies addressing the objectives of each component of EPSDT have offered reliable findings regarding clinical and perhaps cost-effectiveness.[419] These findings have been generated from a prospective study lasting from birth to six years for a three-year birth cohort (2000–2002) of South Carolina children consistently enrolled in Medicaid. These children were part of a 1996 South Carolina Department of Health and Human Services expansion of the state Medicaid system from a single fee-for-service (FFS) health-care plan to a system including a FFS and two separate managed-care models.[420]

These more recent findings are important because, as requested by the AAP more than three decades ago, they narrow the information gap created by lack of empiric findings regarding effectiveness of well-child care.[421] These findings also shed light on the scenario of lack of a medical home, inadequate well-child care, poor health, increased use of hospital emergency departments (EDs) for nonurgent ambulatory care sensitive conditions (ACSCs), and lack of school readiness shared by Medicaid-insured children.[422] Specifically, these findings indicate that many of these egregious outcomes are improved with receipt of EPSDT services in the preschool years.[423]

In the 1996 South Carolina Medicaid health-care model expansion, one added managed-care model was a primary care case management (PCCM) plan, and the second was a health maintenance organization (HMO) model.[424] To optimize policy planning and management, health as reflected by health-service utilization and cost for children enrolled in each model was monitored and compared using secondary data analyses of linked birth certificate, Medicaid claims, and South Carolina K–5 school readiness files.

An early observation was that children enrolled in the two managed-care models had greater utilization of health-care services than those enrolled in the FFS model and that much of this increase was EPSDT and preventive care. It was also noted that children who received the AAP-recommended number of well-child visits in the first year had more cost-efficient care in the second year manifest by receiving fewer nonprimary care provider ACSC ED visits than the children who received fewer EPSDT visits in year one. Based on observations from this six-year prospective cohort study, clinical effectiveness of well-child care was described in four separate publications.[425]

Childhood Hospital Emergency Department (ED) Visits

There are two broad categories of ED visits by children: medical problems preventable with routine primary care or ambulatory care sensitive conditions (ACSCs) and illnesses requiring emergency care.[426] The most commonly reported ACSC ED and hospital admission diagnoses for Medicaid children include asthma; seizures; cellulitis; ear, nose, and throat infections; bacterial pneumonia; kidney and urinary tract infections; and gastrointestinal infections.[427] These diagnoses were monitored in this prospective study.

The parental health education and child preventive care provided during EPSDT visits should limit the occurrence of ACSC illness and enhance parents' ability to distinguish illness requiring ED care from illness requiring an office visit. As such, children with the recommended number of well-child visits should have fewer ED visits for ACSCs than children with fewer than the recommended number. Because ACSC ED visits and sick-child office visits are for similar if not the same diagnoses, the number of ACSC ED visits for children should be inversely proportional to the number of PCP (ACSC) sick-child visits determined by parental choice of health-care location. However, care for an ACSC in an office setting is likely to occur with lower cost than ACSC care in a traditional ED, making the office setting more cost efficient for most ACSC treatment.[428]

The first three reports indicated that when Medicaid-insured children received the recommended well-child care in the first two years of life, expensive ACSC ED visits were fewer, and sick-child (ACSC) PCP visits were increased birth to one, two, and six years as compared to children who received fewer than the recommended number of visits.[429] A fourth report indicated that Medicaid-insured children who received the recommended number of EPSDT visits in the first twenty-four months of life had 23 percent greater odds of being ready for school at the conclusion of the K–5 school year than children with fewer visits in the first two years.[430] Having the recommended preventive-care visits did not affect rates of general ED visits or of hospitalization.

These findings clearly provided evidence for the clinical effectiveness of well-child care. First, receiving the recommended number of EPSDT visits in the first two years of life is associated with a shift in health care from the ED to the PCP office for ACSC diagnoses throughout the first six years of life with increased continuity of care.[431] Second, the fourth publication described the association between receiving the recommended number of well-child visits in the first two years and increased likelihood of school readiness.

Lack of school readiness is a public health concern with adverse psychological, social, and economic consequences for many children insured by Medicaid.[432] Children who are unprepared for school often perform poorly academically, have low self-esteem, and in the long term are at greater risk than others for unemployment, poverty, and crime.[433]

These findings were anticipated based on the expectation that mothers of children with the recommended number of EPSDT visits in the first two years of life receive more guidance from their child's health-care provider about parenting, child health, appropriate health-care utilization, and cognitive development while their children receive more screening and preventive care.[434] Therefore these parents may improve their children's diets, promote physical activity, arrange more social activity, and avoid environmental toxins, all of which may be associated with improved brain development and social skills required for school readiness.[435]

More health screening and preventive care may also improve school readiness by enhancing cognitive development through improved general health. Indeed, immunizations and early treatments of health problems may result in more extended periods of early life spent without illness, fostering the development of cognitive, linguistic, and social skills through more time spent playing and interacting with other children and adults.[436]

Cost-Effectiveness

To assess cost-effectiveness for well-child care in this six-year prospective cohort study, two separate analyses were conducted.[437] The first was to determine if Medicaid–managed care in South Carolina achieved cost containment as compared to the traditional FFS plan in the first two years of life. The hypothesis for this analysis was influenced by the Institute of Medicine (IOM) report indicating that although correcting the underuse of needed health-care services such as EPSDT may improve the quality of care, these corrections often are associated with increased cost.[438] Based on the observed increase in utilization of needed EPSDT services from birth to two years by children enrolled in managed care, the hypothesis tested was that children enrolled in managed care had greater Medicaid costs than children in the FFS plan.[439] Specifically, the analysis compared the Medicaid cost for children continuously enrolled in the PCCM, HMO, or FFS health-care models throughout their first two years of life.

Consistent with the hypothesis, the managed-care-enrolled children with increased EPSDT care had greater Medicaid cost than the FFS enrolled children. The cost for children enrolled in the PCCM model was greater than that for FFS beneficiaries, and the Medicaid cost for HMO enrollees was twice as much as for FFS children and greater than the cost for PCCM beneficiaries. Though managed-care enrollment was associated with increased provision of EPSDT and preventive-care services (and therefore improved quality of care) when compared to that of FFS enrollment, managed care did not contain cost as well as the FFS plan.

A second cost analysis was conducted for the children followed from birth to six years.[440] Although the study children who received the AAP-recommended number of EPSDT and well-child visits in the first two years used fewer ACSC ED visits birth to six years, they also used more EPSDT and sick-child PCP visits than the children with fewer well-child visits. The six-year follow-up findings are similar to the findings for children followed for two years, but these longer-term findings are more instructive because they indicate that the impact of receiving the recommended number of well-child visits in infancy extends beyond the second year and throughout the first six years of life. This shift in location for ACSC care increases PCP continuity of care for children and could indicate more cost-efficient care. However, though reduced use of ACSC ED visits may reflect a Medicaid cost savings, increased EPSDT and sick-child (ACSC) PCP visits both involve cost, and this added cost could offset potential savings from reduced ACSC ED visits. Further, although correcting the underuse of needed health-care services such as EPSDT should enhance the quality of care, such corrections have been reported to increase cost.[441] Therefore, while reduced ACSC ED visits intuitively represent a Medicaid cost savings, the need for a second cost analysis to determine whether cost savings actually occur with receipt of the AAP-recommended number of EPSDT visits was apparent.

In this second cost analysis, the managed-care-enrolled children were excluded due to their small sample size, leaving 18,134 FFS-enrolled study children. The focus for this analysis was the Medicaid cost differences for health-care service use, and more specifically for the nonprimary care provider ACSC ED use from birth to six years for children with the recommended number, and those with fewer than the recommended number of EPSDT visits in the first two years of life. The hypothesis tested was that South Carolina Medicaid children with the AAP-recommended number of EPSDT visits in the first two years of life have a greater total Medicaid cost from birth to six years than children with fewer well-child visits. This hypothesis was again based on the expectation that the cost for increased EPSDT and sick-child PCP visits in the first six years of life for children with the AAP-recommended number of EPSDT visits in the first two years would offset the potential Medicaid cost savings from reduced ACSC ED visits.[442] Consistent with this hypothesis, the children with the AAP-recommended number of EPSDT visits in the first two years of life had a greater (p <0.001) Medicaid cost for health-care services from birth to six years than children with fewer visits.[443] These findings were directly related to the increased PCP EPSDT and sick-child office visits but also to an increased prescription drug Medicaid cost from birth to six years for children with the recommended EPSDT visits in the first two years.

Thus, the more recent findings regarding the clinical and cost-effectiveness of well-child care contribute a much broader understanding than earlier studies regarding how well-child care and the individual components of this preventive care influence the health status of children. These findings are based on large sample sizes of children consistently enrolled in Medicaid from birth to two years (n = 36,662) and from birth to six years (18,134) and compare the health-status outcomes observed among children that received the recommended number of well-child visits with the outcomes observed among those that received fewer visits. Although the immunization component of well-child care has been repeatedly found to reduce child morbidity, these findings suggest that the screening and anticipatory guidance components of well-child care are also associated with improved health status for children.

What Is Quality Care?

The 1990 Institute of Medicine council defined quality of care as "the degree to which health services for individuals and populations increase the likelihood of desired health outcomes."[444]

William B. Pittard III, MD, PhD, MPH

Further, Dr. Darden has clearly noted in chapter 2 of this book that quality health care integrates continuity, a medical home setting, and a continuous, trusted provider. Lastly, in 1948, the World Health Organization clearly established the definition of health as "a state of complete physical, mental, and social wellbeing and not simply the absence of disease or infirmity."[445] Using these definitions with the more recent well-child care findings, one can readily appreciate how receiving the recommended EPSDT services in infancy improves the quality of care for and the health status of children. Both increased ACSC PCP and reduced ACSC ED use with enhanced continuity of care and increased school readiness with improved academic performance and self-esteem for children are associated with receipt of the recommended number of well-child visits in infancy. These associations are clear manifestations of well-child care clinical effectiveness extending throughout the preschool years and perhaps placing children "on track" for life.[446]

Is Well-Child Care a Prudent Investment?

Establishing a quantitative dollar value (cost-effectiveness) for these recently reported qualitative measures of well-child care effectiveness (increased continuity of care and school readiness) is not possible. However, the value of improved physical, mental, and social well-being for the first six years of life and perhaps beyond represents an improved health status of immeasurable value to our children and society. Certainly these data indicate that promotion of preschool well-child care represents a prudent investment in the future of children, our culture, and our nation that has an unquestionably favorable return!

About the Authors

Dr. Pittard received his MD degree from the University of Virginia and is board certified in pediatrics and the sub-board of neonatal-perinatal medicine. He also has a master of public health degree in maternal and child health from the University of Alabama at Birmingham and a PhD in health services and policy management from the University of South Carolina. He has served for more than thirty-five years in academic pediatrics at Case Western Reserve University (1976–1985) and the Medical University of South Carolina (MUSC) (1985–present). For more than fifteen years, he was the director of neonatology at MUSC. He has four children, and his experience and interest in the public health issues of children is reflected by his publications, most recently describing the association between well-child care utilization in the preschool years and both health status and readiness for school by South Carolina Medicaid-insured children.

Dr. Roberts received his MD degree at Texas Tech University Health Sciences Center, completed his residency at the Medical College of Georgia, and did a general pediatric fellowship along with a master of public health in maternal and child health degree at the University of Alabama at Birmingham. He is a professor of pediatrics in the Division of General Pediatrics at the Medical University of South Carolina in Charleston. He is actively involved in patient care, teaching, and clinical investigation. Dr. Roberts is the director of the South Carolina Pediatric Practice Research Network and has coauthored more than forty peer-reviewed publications. On environmental health issues, he is nationally recognized as an expert. Dr. Roberts lives in Daniel Island, South Carolina, and enjoys spending time with his wife and two sons. He is an avid basketball player and ran his first half marathon at age forty-six.

Dr. Gustafson received her MD degree at Southern Illinois University and her master of clinical research at the Medical University of South Carolina, where she is currently an assistant professor of pediatrics. She is the associate pediatric residency program director and the medical director of Pediatric Primary Care, the pediatric continuity clinic. Along with her patient care and teaching roles, her research has involved the use of structured clinical observations with the incorporation of the preventive screening recommendations outlined by Bright Futures/AAP, as well as quality-improvement projects incorporating the CHIPRA quality indicators as part of a patient-centered medical home statewide quality demonstration grant. She lives with her husband, son, and daughter on James Island, South Carolina, and enjoys spending time with her family on the waters surrounding Charleston.

Oscar Lovelace is a board-certified family physician who has been practicing rural family medicine (including obstetrics) since he graduated from residency in 1988 at the University of Virginia, where he served as chief resident. He has served on the SC Board of Family Physicians. Currently he lectures to students at MUSC as a member of the clinical faculty and teaches third-year medical students as part of a required rural clinical rotation. He chaired the SC Governors Health Care Task Force in 2003. In 2011, he was named South Carolina's Family Physician of the Year. In 2012, Dr. Lovelace was among six finalists for the America's Family Physician of the Year award, and in 2015 he was selected as the AAFP National Family Practitioner of the Year. He is married and has four children. His avocation is casting a net for shrimp in the tidal creeks of coastal South Carolina.

Dr. Paul M. Darden joined the department of pediatrics at the Oklahoma University Health Sciences Center in December 2008 as professor of pediatrics, chief of the section of general and community pediatrics, and the CMRI James Paul Linn Chair of Pediatrics. For more than twenty years, he was at the Medical University of South Carolina and held numerous positions. Most recently, he was the director of the South Carolina Pediatric

Practice Research Network (SCPPRN), the director of the Academic Generalist Health Services Research Fellowship, and the vice chair for fellowship programs. His training was in pediatrics at Parkland Hospital and Children's Medical Center in Dallas, followed by fellowship training in epidemiology at McGill and Montréal Children's Hospital, Québec. He has a long-standing interest in the delivery of preventive care and in practice-based research. In Oklahoma, he has been working with Jim Mold and the Oklahoma Physicians Resource/Research Network (OKPRN). Most of his research has related to the delivery of preventive care to children; this has involved numerous studies of the delivery of vaccines and other preventive care in office practice. He has studied continuity of care, dental caries, developmental screening, and obesity among the many issues related to primary care. Currently he is working on a project examining how adolescents and their parents make decisions regarding vaccination and how best to help them with this process.

About the Book

Well-child care is designed to promote optimal health status for children, including school and life success. This preventive care includes anticipatory guidance; continuity of care; assessment of growth and development; screening procedures for vision, hearing, dental, and cognitive development; and immunizations. Anticipatory guidance provides parental health education, counseling, and reassurance. The vast majority of Medicaid-insured children receive fewer than the American Academy of Pediatrics (AAP)–recommended number of well-child visits in the preschool years, and a disproportionate number of children have poor health and lack school readiness. With little empirical data available indicating clinical effectiveness other than for immunizations, the AAP recommendations for well-child care were originally based on consensus expert opinion, and more than three decades later, documentation of effectiveness remained unavailable. This information gap led policy makers to question the value of well-child care and limited incentive to correct its underuse. Only in the last five years have experimental findings indicated an association between well-child care and both more-cost-efficient health care and increased school readiness. Awareness of these findings by insurance company and Medicaid administrators is limited. The purpose for this book is to increase awareness by all stakeholders of the empirically determined clinical effectiveness of well-child care. The short-term goal is to facilitate increased utilization of well-child care, with a longer-term goal of improved child health and life success.

Notes

1. Pittard WB, Hulsey TC, Laditka JN, Laditka SB. Early and Periodic Screening, Diagnosis, and Treatment in Infancy and School Readiness among Children Insured by Medicaid in South Carolina. *Preventing Chronic Disease.* 2012. Available at: http://www.cdc.gov/pcd/issues/2012/11 0333.htm. Accessed: August 18, 2013; and Schor, EL, Abrams M, Shea K. Medicaid: Health Promotion and Disease Prevention for School Readiness. *Health Affairs.* 26, no.2 (2007): 420–429.
2. Social Security Administration. State Innovations in EPSDT. Available at: http://www.ssa.gov/OP_Home/ssact/title19/1905.htm. Accessed: May 4, 2012; Stoddard JJ, St. Peter RF, Newacheck PW. Health Insurance Status and Ambulatory Care for Children. *New England Journal of Medicine* 330 (1994): 1421–1425; and Green M. *The New American Academy of Pediatrics Health-Supervision Guidelines: Implementation and Evaluation, Well-Child Care*, E Charney, ed. Columbus, Ohio: Ross Laboratories, 1986.
3. Committee on Practice and Ambulatory Medicine, Bright Futures Steering Committee. Recommendations for Preventive Pediatric Health Care. *Pediatrics* 120, no. 6 (2007): 1376. http://dx.doi.org/10.1542/peds.2007-2901; and Tanski S, Garfunkel LC, Duncan PM, Weitzman M. Performing Preventive Services: A Bright Futures Handbook. Available at: http://brightfutures.aap.org/continuing_education.html. Accessed May 5, 2012.
4. Raikes H, Pan BA, Luze G, Tamis-LeMonda CS, et al. Mother-Child Bookreading in Low Income Families: Correlates and Outcomes during the First Three Years of Life. *Child Dev* 77, no. 4 (2006): 924–953; Dworkin PH. Ready to Learn: A Mandate for Pediatrics. *J Dev Behav Pediatr* 14, no. 3 (1993): 193–196; and Oja L, Jurimae T. Physical Activity, Motor Ability, and School Readiness of 6-Year Old Children. *Percep Mot Skills* 95, no. 2 (2002): 407–415.
5. Tanski et al. Performing Preventive Services.
6. Lunkenheimer ES, Dishion TJ, Shaw DS, Connell AM, et al. Collateral Benefits of the Family Check-Up on Early Childhood School Readiness: Indirect Effects of Parents' Positive Behavior Support. *Dev Psychol* 44, no. 6 (2008): 1737–1752.
7. Committee on Practice and Ambulatory Medicine. 1376; Telfair J, Kotch JB. The School Age Child from Five to Nine. *Maternal and Child Health.* Kotch JB, ed. Gaithersburg, Maryland: Aspen Publishers, Inc., 1997: 147–171; and Grason H, Morreale M. Health Services for Children and

Adolescents: A Non-System of Care. *Health Care for Children.* Stein REK, ed. New York, United Hospital Fund of New York, 1997: 107–133.

[8] Pittard et al. Early and Periodic Screening; Tanski et al. Performing Preventive Services; and Pittard WB. Well Child Care in Infancy and Emergency Department Use by South Carolina Medicaid Children Birth to Six Years Old. *Southern Medical Journal* 104, no. 8 (2011): 604–608.

[9] Pittard et al. Early and Periodic Screening; Pittard et al. Well Child Care in Infancy. 604–608; and Newacheck PW, Hughes DC, Stoddard JJ. Children's Access to Primary Care: Differences by Race, Income, and Insurance Status. *Pediatrics* 97 (1996): 26–32.

[10] Falik M, Needleman J, Wells BL, Korb J. Ambulatory Care Sensitive Hospitalization and Emergency Visits: Experiences of Medicaid Patients Using Federally Qualified Health Centers. *Med Care* 39 (2001): 551–561.

[11] Pittard WB. Well Child Care in Infancy and Emergency Department Use by South Carolina Medicaid Children Birth to Six Years. *Southern Medical Journal* 104, no. 8 (2011): 604–608; and Starfield B, Shi L. The Medical Home, Access to Care, and Insurance: A Review of Evidence. *Pediatrics* 113, no. 5 (2004): 1493–1498.

[12] Tanski et al. Performing Preventive Services.

[13] Margolis LH, Cole GP, Kotch JB. Historical Foundations of Maternal and Child Health. *Maternal and Child Health.* Kotcj JB, ed. Gaithersburg, Maryland: Aspen Publishers, Inc., 1997: 19–43.

[14] Hutchins VL. A History of Child Health and Pediatrics in the United States. *Health Care for Children.* Stein REK, ed. New York: United Hospital Fund of New York, 1997: 79–106.

[15] Margolis et al. Historical Foundations. 19–43; and Hutchins. A History of Child Health. 79–106.

[16] Margolis et al. Historical Foundations. 19–43; and Schmidt WM, Wallace HM. The Development of Health Services for Mothers and Children in the US. *Maternal and Child Health Practices*, 3rd edition. Wallace HM, Ryan GM, Oglesby A, eds. Oakland: Third Party Publishing Company, 1988.

[17] Veeder BS. *Preventive Pediatrics.* New York: D. Appleton, 1926.

[18] Hutchins. A History of Child Health. 79–106.

[19] Anastasi, A. *Psychological Testing.* New York: Macmillan, 1998: 144; and Baker JP. Women and the Invention of Well Child Care. *Pediatrics* 94, no. 4 (1994): 527–531.

[20] Commission on Medical Education. Second Report. New Haven, CT: Office, Director of the Study, 1928: 57–58; and Aldrich CA. The Composition of Private Practice Pediatrics. *AJDC* 47 (1935): 1051–1064.

[21] Rosenbaum S. Medicaid. *New England Journal of Medicine* 346 (2002): 635–640.

22. Rosenbaum S, Johnson K. Providing Health Care for Low-Income Children: Reconciling Child Health Goals with Child Health Financing Realities. *The Millbank Quarterly* 64 (1980): 442–478.
23. Sardell A, Johnson K. The Politics of EPSDT Policy in the 1990s: Policy Entrepreneurs, Political Streams, and Children's Health Benefits. *The Millbank Quarterly* 76 (1998): 175–205.
24. Rosenbach, M. and Gavin, N. Early and Periodic Screening, Diagnosis, and Treatment and Managed Care. *Annual Review of Public Health* 191 (1998): 507–525; Perkins J, Rivera L, Olson K. National Health Law Program Abigail English and Catherine T. National Center for Youth Law. (1997). EPSDT Update for Child Health Insurance and Medicaid Advocates. Available at: http://www.healthlaw.org/pubs/child1997epsdtupdate.html. Accessed: March 22, 2013; and Rosenbaum S, Proser M, Sonosky C. (2001). Health Policy and Early Child Development: An Overview. Available at: http://www.cmwf.org. Accessed: March 22, 2013.
25. Alpert JJ, Robertson LS, Kosa JK, Heagarty MC, et al. Delivery of Health Care for Children: Report of an Experiment. *Pediatrics* 57, no. 6 (1976): 917–930.
26. Foltz, A. The Development of Ambiguous Federal Policy: Early and Periodic Screening Diagnosis and Treatment (EPSDT). *Millbank Memorial Fund Quarterly/Health and Society* 4 (1975): 35–64; Foltz, A. An Ounce of Prevention: Child Health Policy under Medicaid. Cambridge, Massachusetts: MIT Press, 1982; Thompson, FJ. *Health Policy and the Bureaucracy: Politics and Implementation*. Cambridge, Massachusetts: MIT Press, 1981; and Goggin ML. *Policy Design and the Politics of Implementation: The Case of Child Health Care in the American States*. Knoxville: University of Tennessee Press, 1987.
27. Sardell and Johnson. Politics of EPSDT Policy. 175–205.
28. Ibid.
29. Ibid.; and Sardell A. Child Health Policy in the US: The Paradox of Consensus. *Health Policy and the Disadvantages*. LD Brown, ed. Durham, NC: Duke University Press, 1991.
30. Gavin NI, Adams KI, Herz, EJ, Chawla AJ, et al. The Use of EPSDT and Other Health Care Services by Children Enrolled in Medicaid: The Impact of OBRA '89. *The Millbank Quarterly* 76, no. 2 (1998): 207–250.
31. Rosenbaum S, Shin P, Smith BM, Wehr E, et al. *Negotiating the New Health System: A Nationwide Study of Medicaid Managed-Care Contracts*, Vol 2. Washington, DC: Cent. Health Policy Res., George Washington Univ. Medical Center, 1997.
32. National Health Policy Forum. *State Efforts to Improve Health Care Access for Low Income Children: EPSDT Today and Under Health

Reform. Issue brief no. 639, 1993. Washington, DC: George Washington University.

[33] Sardell and Johnson. Politics of EPSDT Policy. 175–205; and Dewar H, Priest D. Voting Starts in Senate on Health Bill: Republicans Say They Will Not Be Rushed ... Dodd Prenatal Care Amendment Approved. *Washington Post* August 17, 1994: 1.

[34] Sardell and Johnson. Politics of EPSDT Policy. 175–205; and Mann C. Medicaid and the Uninsured: Medicaid and Block Grant Financing Compared. Available at: www.kff.org/Medicaid/upload/Medicaid-and-Block-Grant-Financing-Compared.pdf. Accessed: November 15, 2012.

[35] Mann. Medicaid and the Uninsured; and Ku L, Broaddus M, Wachino V. Medicaid and SCHIP Protected Insurance Coverage for Millions of Low Income Americans. Center on Budget and Policy Procedures, January 31, 2005. Available at: http://www.cbpp.org/cms/?fa=view&id=1013. Accessed: November 19, 2012.

[36] Mann. Medicaid and the Uninsured; and Ramsay C. *US Health Policy Group: Institutional Profiles*. Westport, CT: Greenwood Press, 1995.

[37] Serafini MW. No Strings Attached. *National Journal* May 20, 1995: 1230–34.

[38] Pear R. Governors' Plan to Refit Medicaid Starts to Erode. *New York Times* May 22, 1996: A1, A15.

[39] Sardell and Johnson. Politics of EPSDT Policy. 175–205.

[40] Ibid.

[41] National Health Policy Forum. Restructuring Medicaid: The Governors' Proposal. Testimony before the House Commerce Committee, February 21, 1996. (Same testimony was presented to the Senate Finance Committee.) Washington, DC: George Washington University.

[42] Sardell and Johnson. Politics of EPSDT Policy. 175–205; and Sardell. Child Health Policy.

[43] Rosenbaum S, Johnson K, Sonosky C, Markus A, et al. The Children's Hour: The State Children's Health Insurance Program. *Health Affairs* 17, no. 1 (1998): 75.

[44] Nather D. GOP Divided Over Kid Care Benefits; Choice of Seven Plans under Discussion. Bureau of National Affairs Health Care Policy Report, July 21, 1997: 1120; and Weil A. The New Children's Health Insurance Program: Should States Expand Medicaid? The Urban Institute, Issues and Options for States, series A (October 1997). Washington, DC.

[45] Nather. GOP Divided Over Kid Care. 1120; English A. Expanding Health Insurance for Children and Adolescents: Medicaid or Block Grants? *Youth Law News* (March–April 1997); and Stein REK. *Changing the Lens: Why Focus on Children's Health? Health Care for Children*. Stein REK, ed. New York: United Hospital Fund of New York, 1997: 1–11.

46 Weil. New Children's Health Insurance Program; and English A. Expanding Health Insurance.
47 Gavin et al. Use of EPSDT. 207–250.
48 Sardell and Johnson. Politics of EPSDT Policy. 175–205.
49 Stein. *Changing the Lens.* 1–11.
50 Christakis DA. Continuity of Care: Process or Outcome? *Annals of Family Medicine* 1, no. 3 (September–October 2003): 131–133.
51 American Academy of Pediatrics. American Academy of Pediatrics Ad Hoc Task Force on Definition of the Medical Home: The Medical Home. *Pediatrics* 90, no. 5 (November 1992): 774; Malouin RA, Merten SL. Measuring Medical Homes: Tools to Evaluate the Pediatric Patient- and Family-Centered Medical Home. *Pediatrics AAo, Implementation NCfMH* (2010): 1–43; and Starfield B. What Is Primary Care? *Primary Care: Concepts, Evaluation, and Policy.* New York: Oxford University Press, Inc., 1992: 3–9.
52 American Academy of Pediatrics. The Medical Home. *Pediatrics* 110, no. 1 (Jul 2002): 184–186.
53 American Academy of Family Practice. "Continuity of Care, Definition of." Available at: www.aafp.org/online/en/home/policy/policies/c/continuityofcaredefinition. Accessed: April 17, 2013.
54 American Academy of Pediatrics. The Medical Home. 184–186; and American Academy of Pediatrics. Policy Statement: Organizational Principles to Guide and Define the Child Health Care System and/or Improve the Gealth of All Children. *Pediatrics* 113, no. 5 Suppl (May 2004): 1545–1547.
55 Cabana MD, Jee SH. Does Continuity of Care Improve Patient Outcomes? *The Journal of Family Practice* 53, no. 12 (December 2004): 974–980; and Heagarty MC, Robertson LS, Kosa J, Alpert JJ. Some Comparative Costs in Comprehensive Versus Fragmented Pediatric Care. *Pediatrics* 46, no. 4 (October 1970): 596–603.
56 Heagarty et al. Some Comparative Costs. 596–603; Christakis DA, Mell L, Wright JA, Davis R, Connell FA. The Association between Greater Continuity of Care and Timely Measles-Mumps-Rubella Vaccination. *American Journal of Public Health* 90, no. 6 (June 2000): 962–965; Allred NJ, Wooten KG, Kong Y. The Association of Health Insurance and Continuous Primary Care in the Medical Home on Vaccination Coverage for 19- to 35-Month-Old Children. *Pediatrics* 119, Suppl 1 (February 2007): S4–11; Christakis DA. Does Continuity of Care Matter? Yes: Consistent Contact with a Physician Improves Outcomes. *West J.Med* 175, no. 1 (July 2001): 4; and Smith PJ, Santoli JM, Chu SY, Ochoa DQ, Rodewald LE. The Association between Having a Medical Home and Vaccination Coverage among Children Eligible for the Vaccines for Children Program. *Pediatrics* 116, no. 1 (July 2005): 130–139.

57. Smith et al. Association between Having. 130–139; Cooley WC, McAllister JW, Sherrieb K, Kuhlthau K. Improved Outcomes Associated with Medical Home Implementation in Pediatric Primary Care. *Pediatrics* 124, no. 1 (July 2009): 358–364; and Starfield B. The Medical Home Index Applies Primarily to Children with Special Health Care Needs. *Ambul Pediatr* 4, no. 2 (March–April 2004): 192. author reply 192–193.
58. American Academy of Pediatrics. American Academy of Pediatrics Ad Hoc. 774; Christakis. Does Continuity of Care. 4; and Smith et al. Association between Having. 130–139.
59. Chassin MR, Galvin RW. The Urgent Need to Improve Health Care Quality. *Journal of the American Medical Association* 280 (1998): 1000–1005.
60. Ibid.
61. Lohr KN. *Medicare: A Strategy for Quality Assurance*. Washington, DC: National Academy Press; 1990.
62. Chassin and Galvin. Urgent Need to Improve. 1000–1005.
63. Chassin MR, Kosecoff J, Park RE, et al. Does Inappropriate Use Explain Geographic Variations in the Use of Health Services? A Study of 3 Procedures. *JAMA* 58 (1987): 2533–2537.
64. Early Experiences Matter: Love, Learning, and Routines. National Center for Infants, Toddlers, and Families. Available at: http://main.zerotothree.org/site/PageServer?pagename=ter_key_social_routines. Accessed: March 6, 2013; and Kuo AA, Franke TM, Regalado M, Halfon N. Parent Report of Reading to Young Children. *Pediatrics* 113 (2004): 1944–1951.
65. Theilheimer R. Molding to the Children: Primary Caregiving and Continuity of Care. *Zero to Three Bulletin* 26, no. 3 (January 2006): 50–56.
66. Howes C, Hamilton CE. The Changing Experience of Child Care: Changes in Teachers and in Teacher-Child Relationships and Children's Social Competence with Peers. *Early Childhood Research Quarterly* 8, no. 1 (1993): 15–32.
67. Cryer D, Hurwitz S, Wilery M. Continuity of Caregiver for Infants and Toddlers. Available at: http://ecap.crc.illinois.edu/eecearchive/digests/2003/cryer03.html. Accessed April 17, 2013; and Lecture on Primary Caregiving, Continuity of Care, and Small Group Size. Available at: www.vvc.edu/academic/child_development/sypkens/ht/course1/faculty/cd11lectweek8a.html. Accessed: April 17, 2013.
68. American Academy of Family Practice. "Continuity of Care."
69. Ibid.; Inkelas M, Schuster MM, Olson LM, Park CM, Halfon N. Continuity of Primary Care Clinician in Early Childhood. *Pediatrics* 113 (2004): 1914–1925; and The Ounce of Prevention, and Why Investments in Early Childhood Work. Available at: http://www.ounceofprevention.org/

about/why-early-childhood-investments-work.php. Accessed: April 17, 2013.
70 Inkelas et al. Continuity of Primary Care. 1914–1925.
71 Gulliford M, Naithari S, Morgan M. "What Is Continuity of Care?" *J Health Serv Res Policy* 11, no. 4 (2006): 248–50.
72 Heagarty et al. Some Comparative Costs. 596–603; Alpert JJ, Robertson LS, Kosa J, Heagarty MC, Haggerty RJ. Delivery of Health Care for Children: Report of an Experiment. *Pediatrics* 57, no. 6 (June 1976): 917–930; Christakis DA, Wright JA, Zimmerman FJ, Bassett AL, Connell FA. Continuity of Care Is Associated with Well-Coordinated Care. *Ambul Pediatr* 3, no. 2 (March–April 2003): 82–86; Christakis DA, Mell L, Koepsell TD, Zimmerman FJ, Connell FA. Association of Lower Continuity of Care with Greater Risk of Emergency Department Use and Hospitalization in Children. *Pediatrics* 107, no. 3 (March 2001): 524–529; Christakis DA, Wright JA, Koepsell TD, Emerson S, Connell FA. Is Greater Continuity of Care Associated with Less Emergency Department Utilization? *Pediatrics* 103, no. 4 Pt. 1 (April 1999): 738–742; Dietrich AJ, Marton KI. Does Continuous Care from a Physician Make a Difference? *J. Fam. Pract.* 15, no. 5 (November 1982): 929–937; Garrison WT, Bailey EN, Garb J, Ecker B, Spencer P, Sigelman D. Interactions between Parents and Pediatric Primary Care Physicians about Children's Mental Health. *Hosp. Community Psychiatry* 43, no. 5 (May 1992): 489–493; Lewis C. What is the evidence? *Am. J. Dis. Child* 122, no. 6 (December 1971): 469–474; Lochman JE. Factors Related to Patients' Satisfaction with Their Medical Care. *J. Community Health* 9, no. 2 (1983): 91–109; McCune YD, Richardson MM, Powell JA. Psychosocial Health Issues in Pediatric Practices: Parents' Knowledge and Concerns. *Pediatrics* 74, no. 2 (August 1984): 183–190; and Weiss GL, Ramsey CA. Regular Source of Primary Medical Care and Patient Satisfaction. *QRB Qual. Rev. Bull.* 15, no. 6 (June 1989): 180–184.
73 McCune et al. Psychosocial Health Issues. 183–190; Weiss and Ramsey. Regular Source of Primary Medical Care. 180–184; Forrest CB, Starfield B. The Effect of First-Contact Care with Primary Care Clinicians on Ambulatory Health Care Expenditures. *The Journal of Family Practice* 43, no. 1 (July 1996): 40–48; and De Maeseneer JM, De Prins L, Gosset C, Heyerick J. Provider Continuity in Family Medicine: Does It Make a Difference for Total Health Care Costs? *Annals of Family Medicine* 1, no. 3 (September–October 2003): 144–148.
74 Yawn BP, Yawn RA, Geier GR, Xia Z, Jacobsen SJ. The Impact of Requiring Patient Authorization for Use of Data in Medical Records Research. *The Journal of Family Practice* 47, no. 5 (November 1998): 361–365.
75 Feikema SM, Klevens RM, Washington ML, Barker L. Extraimmunization among US Children. *Journal of the American Medical Association*

283, no. 10 (March 8, 2000): 1311–1317; Davis RL. Vaccine Extraimmunization—Too Much of a Good Thing? *JAMA* 283, no. 10 (March 8, 2000): 1339–1340; Mell LK, Davis RL, Mullooly JP, et al. Polio Extraimmunization in Children Younger Than Two Years after Changes in Immunization Recommendations. *Pediatrics* 111, no. 2 (February 2003): 296–301; Strine TW, Barker LE, Jain RB, Washington ML, Chu SY, Mokdad AH. Extraimmunization in Children through 2000. *Journal of the American Medical Association* 287, no. 5 (February 6, 2002): 588–589; and Rabo E. Risk of Overvaccination against Tetanus—Who Is Deciding: The National Board of Health and Welfare or the Manufacturer? *Lakartidningen* 86, no. 8 (February 22, 1989): 615–616.

[76] Mainz J. Defining and Classifying Clinical Indicators for Quality Improvement. *Int J Qual Health Care* 15, no. 6 (December 2003): 523–530.

[77] Committee on Practice and Ambulatory Medicine, Bright Futures Steering Committee. Recommendations for Preventive Pediatric Health Care. *Pediatrics* 120, no. 6 (2007): 1376. http://dx.doi.org/10.1542/peds.2007-2901; Gavin NI, Adams EK, Hertz EJ, Chawla AJ, et al. The Use of EPSDT and Other Healthcare Services by Children Enrolled in Medicaid: The Impact of OBRA '89. *Milbank Quarterly* 76, no. 2 (1998): 207–232; Grason H, Morreale M. Health Services for Children and Adolescents: A "Non-System" of Care. *Health Care for Children: What's Right, What's Wrong, and What's Next.* Stein REK and Brookes P, eds. New York: United Hospital Fund, 1997; Farel AM and Kotch JB. The Child from One to Four: The Toddler and Preschool Years. *Maternal and Child Health: Programs, Problems, and Policy in Public Health.* Kotch JB, ed. Gaithersburg, MD: Aspen Publications, 1997.

[78] American Academy of Family Practice. "Continuity of Care"; and Romaire MA, Bell JF, Grossman DC. Health Care Use and Expenditures Associated with Access to the Medical Home for Children and Youth. *Medical Care* 50 (2012): 262–269.

[79] Christakis. Association between Greater Continuity. 962–965; US Congress, Office of Technology Assessment, Healthy Children: Investing in the Future, chapter 6, pages 119–144, OTA-H-345. Washington, DC: US Government Printing Office, February 1988; Breslau N, Haug M. Service Delivery Structure and Continuity of Care: A Case Study of a Pediatric Practice in Process of Reorganization. *J Health and Social Behavior* 17 (1976): 339–352; and Brezlau N, Reeb K. Continuity of Care in a University-Based Practice. *J Medical Educ* 50 (1975): 965–969.

[80] Starfield BS, Shi L. The Medical Home, Access to Care, and Insurance: A Review of Evidence. *Pediatrics* 113, no. 5 (2004): 1493–1498; and Brousseau DC, Meurer JR, Isenberg ML, Association between Infant

Continuity of Care and Pediatric Emergency Department Utilization. *Pediatrics* 113, no. 4 (2004): 738–741.

[81] US Congress, Office of Technology Assessment. Healthy Children. 119–144.

[82] Pittard W, Laditka J, and Laditka S. Associations between Early and Periodic Screening, Diagnosis, and Treatment and Health Outcomes among Medicaid Insured Infants in South Carolina. *J. Pediatrics* 151 (2007): 414–418; Pittard, William B. Well Child Care in Infancy and Emergency Department Use by South Carolina Medicaid Children Birth to Six Years Old. *Southern Medical Journal* 104, no. 8 (2011): 604–608; and Pittard WB, Hulsey, TC, Laditka JN, Laditka SB. School Readiness Among Children Insured by Medicaid in South Carolina. *Preventing Chronic Disease*. 2012: Available at: http://www.cdc.gov/pcd/issuesl2012/11_0333.htm.

[83] Tom JD, Tseng CW, Davis J, Solomon C, Zhou C, Mangione-Smith R. Missed Well-Child Care Visits, Low Continuity of Care, and Risk of Ambulatory Care Sensitive Hospitalizations in Young Children. *Arch Pediatr Adolesc Med* 164, no. 11 (2010): 1052–1058.

[84] Bice TW, Boxerman SB. A Quantitative Measure of Continuity of Care. *Med Care* 15, no. 4 (1977): 347–349.

[85] American Academy of Pediatrics. *Bright Futures: Guidelines for Health Supervision of Infants, Children, and Adolescents*, third edition. Elk Grove Village, IL: American Academy of Pediatrics, 2008.

[86] Therrell BL, Jr., Berenbaum SA, Manter-Kapanke V, et al. Results of screening 1.9 Million Texas Newborns for 21-Hydroxylase-Deficient Congenital Adrenal Hyperplasia. *Pediatrics* 101 (1998): 583–90; and Varness TS, Allen DB, Hoffman GL. Newborn Screening for Congenital Adrenal Hyperplasia Has Reduced Sensitivity in Girls. *The Journal of Pediatrics* 147 (2005): 493–98.

[87] US Preventive Services Task Force. Universal Screening for Hearing Loss in Newborns: US Preventive Services Task Force Recommendation Statement. *Pediatrics* 122 (2008): 143–48.

[88] Mehl AL, Thomson V. The Colorado Newborn Hearing Screening Project, 1992–1999: On the Threshold of Effective Population-Based Universal Newborn Hearing Screening. *Pediatrics* 109 (2002): E7.

[89] Gifford KA, Holmes MG, Bernstein HH. Hearing Loss in Children. *Pediatrics in Review / American Academy of Pediatrics* 30 (2009): 207–15.

[90] US Preventive Services Task Force. Universal Screening. 143–48.

[91] Casselbrant ML, Brostoff LM, Cantekin EI, et al. Otitis Media with Effusion in Preschool Children. *The Laryngoscope* 95 (1985): 428–36; Casselbrant ML, Furman JM, Rubenstein E, Mandel EM. Effect of Otitis Media on the Vestibular System in Children. *The Annals of Otology,*

Rhinology, and Laryngology 104 (1995): 620–24; Fiellau-Nikolasjen M. Tympanometry and Secretory Otitis Media. Observations on Diagnosis, Epidemiology, Treatment and Prevention in Prospective Cohort Studies of Three-Year-Old Children [thesis]. Acta Otolaryngologica Stockholm 394 (1983): 1–73; and Teele DW, Klein JO, Rosner B. Epidemiology of Otitis Media during the First Seven Years of Life in Children in Greater Boston: A Prospective, Cohort Study. The Journal of Infectious Diseases 160 (1989): 83–94.

[92] Wessex Universal Neonatal Hearing Screening Trial Group. Controlled Trial of Universal Neonatal Screening for Early Identification of Permanent Childhood Hearing Impairment. Lancet 352 (1998): 1957–64.

[93] US Preventive Services Task Force. Universal Screening. 143–48.

[94] Harrison RV, Gordon KA, Mount RJ. Is There a Critical Period for Cochlear Implantation in Congenitally Deaf Children? Analyses of Hearing and Speech Perception Performance after Implantation. Developmental Psychobiology 46 (2005): 252–61.

[95] Korver AM, Konings S, Dekker FW, et al. Newborn hearing screening versus Later Hearing Screening and Developmental Outcomes in Children with Permanent Childhood Hearing Impairment. The Journal of the American Medical Association 304 (2010): 1701–18.

[96] Rosenfeld RM, Jang DW, Tarashansky K. Tympanostomy Tube Outcomes in Children At-Risk and Not At-Risk for Developmental Delays. International Journal of Pediatric Otorhinolaryngology 75 (2011): 190–95.

[97] Paradise JL, Feldman HM, Campbell TF, et al. Effect of Early or Delayed Insertion of Tympanostomy Tubes for Persistent Otitis Media on Developmental Outcomes at the Age of Three Years. The New England Journal of Medicine 344 (2001): 1179–87; Paradise JL, Campbell TF, Dollaghan CA, et al. Developmental Outcomes after Early or Delayed Insertion of Tympanostomy Tubes. The New England Journal of Medicine 353 (2005): 576–86; and Paradise JL, Feldman HM, Campbell TF, et al. Tympanostomy Tubes and Developmental Outcomes at 9 to 11 Years of Age. The New England Journal of Medicine 356 (2007): 248–61.

[98] Tingley, Donald H. Vision Screening Essentials: Screening Today for Eye Disorders in the Pediatric Patient. Pediatrics in Review 28 (2007): 54–61.

[99] Pollard ZF, Manley D. Long-term Results in the Treatment of Unilateral High Myopia with Amblyopia. American Journal of Ophthalmology 78 (1974): 397–99; and US Department of Health, Education, and Welfare. Eye Examination Findings among Youths Aged 12–17 Years, United States. DHEW Publication No 76-1637 (1976): 11.

[100] Mark H, Mark T. Parental Reasons for Non-Response Following a Referral in School Vision Screening. *The Journal of School Health* 69 (1999): 35–38; and Preslan MW, Novak A. Baltimore Vision Screening Project: Phase 2. *Ophthalmology* 105 (1998): 150–53.

[101] Manny RE, Sinnott LT, Jones-Jordan LA, et al. Predictors of Adequate Correction Following Vision Screening Failure. *Optometry and Vision Science: Official Publication of the American Academy of Optometry* 89 (2012): 892–900.

[102] Campbell LR, Charney E. Factors Associated with Delay in Diagnosis of Childhood Amblyopia. *Pediatrics* 87 (1991): 178–85.

[103] US Preventive Services Task Force. Vision Screening for Children 1 to 5 Years of Age: US Preventive Services Task Force Recommendation Statement. *Pediatrics* 127 (2011): 340–46.

[104] Council on Children with Disabilities, Section on Developmental Behavioral Pediatrics, Bright Futures Steering Committee, Medical Home Initiatives for Children with Special Needs Project Advisory Committee. Identifying Infants and Young Children with Developmental Disorders in the Medical Home: An Algorithm for Developmental Surveillance and Screening. *Pediatrics* 118 (2006): 405–20.

[105] Radecki L, Sand-Loud N, O'Connor KG, Sharp S, Olson LM. Trends in the Use of Standardized Tools for Developmental Screening in Early Childhood: 2002–2009. *Pediatrics* 128 (2011): 14–19.

[106] Committee on Children with Disabilities. Developmental Surveillance and Screening of Infants and Young Children. *Pediatrics* 108 (2001): 192–96.

[107] Council on Children with Disabilities. Identifying Infants. 405–20.

[108] Marks KP, LaRosa AC. Understanding Developmental-Behavioral Screening Measures. *Pediatrics in Review / American Academy of Pediatrics* 33 (2012): 448–57; quiz 57–58.

[109] Shevell M, Ashwal S, Donley D, et al. Practice Parameter: Evaluation of the Child with Global Developmental Delay: Report of the Quality Standards Subcommittee of the American Academy of Neurology and the Practice Committee of the Child Neurology Society. *Neurology* 60 (2003): 367–80.

[110] Shevell MI, Majnemer A, Rosenbaum P, Abrahamowicz M. Etiologic Determination of Childhood Developmental Delay. *Brain Dev* 23 (2001): 228–35.

[111] Council on Children with Disabilities. Identifying Infants. 405–20.

[112] Nelson HD, Nygren P, Walker M, Panoscha R. Screening for Speech and Language Delay in Preschool Children: Systematic Evidence Review for the US Preventive Services Task Force. *Pediatrics* 117 (2006): e298–319; and National Research Council. *Educating Children with Autism*. Washington, DC: The National Academy Press, 2001.

113 Stone WL, Lee EB, Ashford L, et al. Can Autism Be Diagnosed Accurately in Children Under 3 Years? *Journal of Child Psychology and Psychiatry, and Allied Disciplines* 40 (1999): 219–26.

114 Johnson CP. Recognition of Autism before Age 2 Years. *Pediatrics in Review / American Academy of Pediatrics* 29 (2008): 86–96.

115 Wiggins LD, Baio J, Rice C. Examination of the Time between First Evaluation and First Autism Spectrum Diagnosis in a Population-Based Sample. *Journal of Developmental and Behavioral Pediatrics* 27 (2006): S79–87.

116 Johnson CP, Myers SM, Disabilities at CoCW. Identification and Evaluation of Children with Autism Spectrum Disorders. *Pediatrics* 120 (2007): 1183–215.

117 Robins DL, Fein D, Barton ML, Green JA. The Modified Checklist for Autism in Toddlers: An Initial Study Investigating the Early Detection of Autism and Pervasive Developmental Disorders. *Journal of Autism and Developmental Disorders* 31 (2001): 131–44.

118 Gupta VB, Hyman SL, Johnson CP, et al. Identifying Children with Autism Early? *Pediatrics* 119 (2007): 152–53.

119 Autism and Developmental Disabilities Monitoring Network Surveillance Year Principal Investigators, Centers for Disease Control and Prevention. Prevalence of Autism Spectrum Disorders—Autism and Developmental Disabilities Monitoring Network, 14 Sites, United States, 2008. *Morbidity and Mortality Weekly Report Surveillance Summaries* 61 (2012): 1–19.

120 Rosenberg RE, Law JK, Yenokyan G, McGready J, Kaufmann WE, Law PA. Characteristics and Concordance of Autism Spectrum Disorders among 277 Twin Pairs. *Arch Pediatr Adolesc Med* 163 (2009): 907–14; Ozonoff S, Young GS, Carter A, et al. Recurrence Risk for Autism Spectrum Disorders: A Baby Siblings Research Consortium Study. *Pediatrics* 128 (2011): e488–95; and Cohen D, Pichard N, Tordjman S, et al. Specific Genetic Disorders and Autism: Clinical Contribution towards Their Identification. *Journal of Autism and Developmental Disorders* 35 (2005): 103–16.

121 Eaves LC, Ho HH. Brief Report: Stability and Change in Cognitive and Behavioral Characteristics of Autism through Childhood. *Journal of Autism and Developmental Disorders* 26 (1996): 557–69; Eaves LC, Ho HH. The Very Early Identification of Autism: Outcome to Age 4.5–5. *Journal of Autism and Developmental Disorders* 34 (2004): 367–78; and Harris SL, Handleman JS. Age and IQ at Intake as Predictors of Placement for Young Children with Autism: A Four- to Six-year Follow-up. *Journal of Autism and Developmental Disorders* 30 (2000): 137–42.

122 Kleinman JM, Robins DL, Ventola PE, et al. The Modified Checklist for Autism in Toddlers: A Follow-up Study Investigating the Early Detection

of Autism Spectrum Disorders. *Journal of Autism and Developmental Disorders* 38 (2008): 827–39; and Dumont-Mathieu T, Fein D. Screening for Autism in Young Children: The Modified Checklist for Autism in Toddlers (M-CHAT) and Other Measures. *Mental Retardation and Developmental Disabilities Research Reviews* 11 (2005): 253–62.

[123] Committee on Children with Disabilities. American Academy of Pediatrics: The Pediatrician's Role in the Diagnosis and Management of Autistic Spectrum Disorder in Children. *Pediatrics* 107 (2001): 1221–26.

[124] Ibid.

[125] Centers for Disease Control and Prevention. Increased lead absorption and Lead Poisoning in Young Children: A Statement by the Center for Disease Control. *The Journal of Pediatrics* 87 (1975): 824–30.

[126] Centers for Disease Control and Prevention. Preventing Lead Poisoning in Young Children. A Statement by the Centers for Disease Control. US Department of Health and Human Services, Public Health Service, 1991.

[127] Bellinger DC, Stiles KM, Needleman HL. Low-level Lead Exposure, Intelligence and Academic Achievement: A Long-term Follow-up Study. *Pediatrics* 90 (1992): 855–61; Dietrich KN, Succop PA, Berger OG, Keith RW. Lead Exposure and the Central Auditory Processing Abilities and Cognitive Development of Urban Children: The Cincinnati Lead Study Cohort at Age 5 Years. *Neurotoxicology and Teratology* 14 (1992): 51–56; and Needleman HL, Gunnoe C, Leviton A, et al. Deficits in Psychologic and Classroom Performance of Children with Elevated Dentine Lead Levels. *The New England Journal of Medicine* 300 (1979): 689–95.

[128] Centers for Disease Control and Prevention. Preventing Lead Poisoning.

[129] Canfield RL, Henderson CR, Jr., Cory-Slechta DA, Cox C, Jusko TA, Lanphear BP. Intellectual Impairment in Children with Blood Lead Concentrations below 10 microg per Deciliter. *The New England Journal of Medicine* 348 (2003): 1517–26; Jusko TA, Henderson CR, Lanphear BP, Cory-Slechta DA, Parsons PJ, Canfield RL. Blood Lead Concentrations <10 microg/dL and Child Intelligence at 6 Years of Age. *Environmental Health Perspectives* 116 (2008): 243–48; and Braun JM, Kahn RS, Froehlich T, Auinger P, Lanphear BP. Exposures to Environmental Toxicants and Attention Deficit Hyperactivity Disorder in US Children. *Environmental Health Perspectives* 114 (2006): 1904–1909.

[130] Centers for Disease Control and Prevention. Low Level Lead Exposure Harms Children: A Renewed Call for Primary Prevention. A Report of the Advisory Committee on Childhood Lead Poisoning Prevention of the Centers for Disease Control and Prevention, January 2012.

[131] Committee on Children with Disabilities. American Academy of Pediatrics. 1221–26; and Centers for Disease Control and Prevention. Low Level Lead Exposure.

[132] Centers for Disease Control and Prevention. Low Level Lead Exposure; and Centers for Disease Control and Prevention. Screening Young Children for Lead Poisoning: Guidance for State and Local Public Health Officials. Atlanta: CDC, 1997.

[133] Schwab LT, Roberts JR, Reigart JR. Inaccuracy in Parental Reporting of the Age of Their Home for Lead-screening Purposes. *Arch Pediatr Adolesc Med* 157 (2003): 584–86.

[134] Centers for Disease Control and Prevention. Update: Blood Lead Levels—United States, 1991–1994. *Morbidity and Mortality Weekly Report* 46 (1997): 141–46.

[135] Centers for Disease Control and Prevention. Blood Lead Levels—United States, 1999–2002. *Morbidity and Mortality Weekly Report* 54 (2005): 513–16.

[136] Jones RL, Homa DM, Meyer PA, et al. Trends in Blood Lead Levels and Blood Lead Testing among US Children Aged 1 to 5 Years, 1988–2004. *Pediatrics* 123 (2009): e376–85.

[137] Roberts JR, Hulsey TC, Curtis GB, Reigart JR. Using Geographic Information Systems to Assess Risk for Elevated Blood Lead Levels in Children. *Public Health Reports* 118 (2003): 221–29; and Dignam TA, Evens A, Eduardo E, et al. High-intensity Targeted Screening for Elevated Blood Lead Levels among Children in 2 Inner-city Chicago Communities. *American Journal of Public Health* 94 (2004): 1945–51.

[138] Centers for Disease Control and Prevention. Low Level Lead Exposure.

[139] Chisolm JJ, Jr. The Use of Chelating Agents in the Treatment of Acute and Chronic Lead Intoxication in Childhood. *The Journal of Pediatrics* 73 (1969): 1–38; and Chisolm JJ, Jr., Harrison HE. The Treatment of Acute Lead Encephalopathy in Children. *Pediatrics* 19 (1957): 2–20.

[140] Chisolm Jr. Use of Chelating Agents. 1–38; Chisolm Jr. et al. Treatment of Acute. 2–20; and Chisolm JJ, Jr. Treatment of Acute Lead Intoxication—Choice of Chelating Agents and Supportive Therapeutic Measures. *Clinical Toxicology* 3 (1970): 527–40.

[141] Whitlock NH. Reigart JR. Priester LE. Lead Poisoning in South Carolina. *Journal of the South Carolina Medical Association* 73, no. 8 (1977): 378–80.

[142] Centers for Disease Control and Prevention. Preventing Lead Poisoning.

[143] Centers for Disease Control and Prevention. Screening Young Children.

[144] Jones et al. Trends in Blood Lead. e376–85.

[145] Centers for Disease Control and Prevention. Blood Lead Levels. 513–16; and Jones et al. Trends in Blood Lead. e376–85.

[146] Jones et al. Trends in Blood Lead. e376–85.

[147] Roberts JR, Allen CL, Ligon C, Reigart JR. Are Children Still at Risk for Lead Poisoning? *Clinical Pediatrics* 52 (2013): 125–130.

[148] Baker RD, Greer FR, The Nutrition Committee Diagnosis and Prevention of Iron Deficiency and Iron-Deficiency Anemia in Infants and Young Children (0–3 Years of Age). *Pediatrics* 126 (2010): 1040–50.

[149] Ibid.

[150] McCann JC, Ames BN. An Overview of Evidence for a Causal Relation between Iron Deficiency during Development and Deficits in Cognitive or Behavioral Function. *The American Journal of Clinical Nutrition* 85 (2007): 931–45.

[151] Baker et al. Diagnosis and Prevention. 1040–50; McCann and Ames. Overview of Evidence. 931–45; and Grantham-McGregor S, Ani C. A Review of Studies on the Effect of Iron Deficiency on Cognitive Development in Children. *The Journal of Nutrition* 131 (2001): 649S–68S.

[152] American Academy of Pediatrics Committee on Infectious Diseases. Red Book: 2012 Report of the Committee on Infectious Diseases, 29th edition, 2012.

[153] American Academy of Pediatrics. Red Book; and Pediatric Tuberculosis Collaborative Group. Targeted Tuberculin Skin Testing and Treatment of Latent Tuberculosis Infection in Children and Adolescents. *Pediatrics* 114 (2004): 1175–201.

[154] American Academy of Pediatrics. Red Book; Pediatric Tuberculosis Collaborative. Targeted Tuberculin Skin Testing. 1175–201; and Ozuah PO, Ozuah TP, Stein RE, Burton W, Mulvihill M. Evaluation of a Risk Assessment Questionnaire Used to Target Tuberculin Skin Testing in Children. *JAMA* 285 (2001): 451–53.

[155] Froehlich H, Ackerson LM, Morozumi PA, Pediatric Tuberculosis Study Group of Kaiser Permanente, Northern California. Targeted Testing of Children for Tuberculosis: Validation of a Risk Assessment Questionnaire. *Pediatrics* 107 (2001): E54; and Centers for Disease Control and Prevention. Targeted Tuberculin Testing and Treatment of Latent Tuberculosis Infection. American Thoracic Society. Recommendations and Reports from Centers for Disease Control. *Morbidity and Mortality Weekly Report* 49 (2000): 1–51.

[156] American Academy of Pediatrics. Red Book.

[157] Froehlich et al. Targeted Testing. E54.

[158] Ibid.

[159] Freeman RJ, Mancuso JD, Riddle MS, Keep LW. Systematic Review and Meta-analysis of TST Conversion Risk in Deployed Military and Long-term Civilian Travelers. *Journal of Travel Medicine* 17 (2010): 233–42.

[160] Flaherman VJ, Porco TC, Marseille E, Royce SE. Cost-effectiveness of Alternative Strategies for Tuberculosis Screening before Kindergarten Entry. *Pediatrics* 120 (2007): 90–99.

[161] Ibid.

[162] Halfon N, Verhoef PA, Kuo AA. Childhood Antecedents to Adult Cardiovascular Disease. *Pediatrics in Review / American Academy of Pediatrics* 33 (2012): 51–60; quiz 1.

[163] National High Blood Pressure Education Program Working Group on High Blood Pressure in Children and Adolescents. The Fourth Report on the Diagnosis, Evaluation, and Treatment of High Blood Pressure in Children and Adolescents. *Pediatrics* 114 (2004): 555–76.

[164] Expert Panel on Integrated Guidelines for Cardiovascular Health and Risk Reduction in Children and Adolescents, National Heart, Lung, and Blood Institute. Expert Panel on Integrated Guidelines for Cardiovascular Health and Risk Reduction in Children and Adolescents: Summary Report. *Pediatrics* 128 Supplement 5 (2011): S213–56.

[165] National High Blood Pressure Education Program. Fourth Report. 555–76.

[166] Expert Panel on Integrated Guidelines. Summary Report. S213–56.

[167] American Academy of Pediatrics. *Bright Futures*.

[168] Sorof JM. Prevalence and Consequence of Systolic Hypertension in Children. *American Journal of Hypertension* 15 (2002): 57S–60S; McNiece KL, Poffenbarger TS, Turner JL, Franco KD, Sorof JM, Portman RJ. Prevalence of Hypertension and Pre-hypertension among Adolescents. *The Journal of Pediatrics* 150, no.6 (2007): e640–e644; Muntner P, He J, Cutler JA, Wildman RP, Whelton PK. Trends in Blood Pressure among Children and Adolescents. *JAMA* 291 (2004): 2107–13; and Din-Dzietham R, Liu Y, Bielo MV, Shamsa F. High Blood Pressure Trends in Children and Adolescents in National Surveys, 1963–2002. *Circulation* 116 (2007): 1488–96.

[169] Expert Panel on Integrated Guidelines. Summary Report. S213–56.

[170] Mitsnefes MM. Hypertension in Children and Adolescents. *Pediatric Clinics of North America* 53 (2006): VIII 493–512; and Sugiyama T, Xie D, Graham-Maar RC, Inoue K, Kobayashi Y, Stettler N. Dietary and Lifestyle Factors Associated with Blood Pressure among US Adolescents. *The Journal of Adolescent Health* 40 (2007): 166–72.

[171] US Preventive Services Task Force. Screening for High Blood Pressure: Recommendations and Rationale. *American Family Physician* 68 (2003): 2019–22.

[172] Sun SS, Grave GD, Siervogel RM, Pickoff AA, Arslanian SS, Daniels SR. Systolic Blood Pressure in Childhood Predicts Hypertension and Metabolic Syndrome Later in Life. *Pediatrics* 119 (2007): 237–46; and Erlingsdottir A, Indridason OS, Thorvaldsson O, Edvardsson VO. Blood Pressure in Children and Target-organ Damage Later in Life. *Pediatric Nephrology* 25 (2010): 323–28.

[173] Chen X, Wang Y. Tracking of Blood Pressure from Childhood to Adulthood: A Systematic Review and Meta-regression Analysis. *Circulation* 117 (2008): 3171–80.

[174] Brady TM, Fivush B, Flynn JT, Parekh R. Ability of Blood Pressure to Predict Left Ventricular Hypertrophy in Children with Primary Hypertension. *The Journal of Pediatrics* 152. (2008): e73–e78.

[175] Barlow SE, Expert Committee. Expert Committee Recommendations Regarding the Prevention, Assessment, and Treatment of Child and Adolescent Overweight and Obesity: Summary Report. *Pediatrics* 120, Suppl 4 (2007): S164–92; and Ogden C, Caroll M, Division of Health and Nutrition and Examination Surveys. Prevalence of Obesity among Children and Adolescents, Trends 1963–1965 through 2007–2008. CDC National Center for Health Statistics, 2010.

[176] Hammer LD, Kraemer HC, Wilson DM, Ritter PL, Dornbusch SM. Standardized Percentile Curves of Body-mass Index for Children and Adolescents. *American Journal of Diseases of Children* 145 (1991): 259–63; and Must A, Dallal GE, Dietz WH. Reference Data for Obesity: 85th and 95th Percentiles of Body Mass Index (wt/ht^2) and Triceps Skinfold Thickness. *The American Journal of Clinical Nutrition* 53 (1991): 839–46.

[177] Krebs NF, Jacobson MS, American Academy of Pediatrics Committee on Nutrition. Prevention of Pediatric Overweight and Obesity. *Pediatrics* 112 (2003): 424–30; and American Academy of Pediatrics. AAP Publications Retired or Reaffirmed, October 2006. *Pediatrics* 119 (2007): 405.

[178] American Academy of Pediatrics. AAP Publications. 405.

[179] Ogden and Caroll. Prevalence of Obesity.

[180] Freedman DS, Mei Z, Srinivasan SR, Berenson GS, Dietz WH. Cardiovascular Risk Factors and Excess Adiposity among Overweight Children and Adolescents: the Bogalusa Heart Study. *The Journal of Pediatrics* 150 (2007): 12–7e2.

[181] Whitlock EP, Williams SB, Gold R, Smith PR, Shipman SA. Screening and Interventions for Childhood Overweight: A Summary of Evidence for the US Preventive Services Task Force. *Pediatrics* 116 (2005): e125–e44.

[182] Freedman et al. Cardiovascular Risk Factors. 12–7e2; and Whitlock et al. Screening and Interventions. e125–e44.

[183] Han JC, Lawlor DA, Kimm SY. Childhood Obesity. *Lancet* 375 (2010): 1737–48; and Sutherland ER. Obesity and Asthma. *Immunology and Allergy Clinics of North America* 28 (2008): IX 589–602.

[184] Han et al. Childhood Obesity. 1737–48; Sutherland. Obesity and Asthma. 589–602; Biro FM, Wien M. Childhood Obesity and Adult Morbidities. *The American Journal of Clinical Nutrition* 91 (2010): 1499S–1505S; Whitaker RC, Wright JA, Pepe MS, Seidel KD, Dietz WH. Predicting

Obesity in Young Adulthood from Childhood and Parental Obesity. *The New England Journal of Medicine* 337 (1997): 869–73; and Serdula MK, Ivery D, Coates RJ, Freedman DS, Williamson DF, Byers T. Do Obese Children Become Obese Adults? A Review of the Literature. *Preventive Medicine* 22 (1993): 167–77.

[185] NHLBI Obesity Education Initiative Expert Panel on the Identification, Evaluation, and Treatment of Obesity in Adults (US). *Clinical Guidelines on the Identification, Evaluation, and Treatment of Overweight and Obesity in Adults: The Evidence Report.* Bethesda, MD: National Heart, Lung, and Blood Institute, 1998.

[186] National Center for Health Statistics. Health, United States, 1998, with Socioeconomic Status and Health Chartbook. Hyattsville, MD: National Center for Health Statistics, 1998.

[187] Stein REK. Changing the Lens: Why Focus on Children's Health. *Health Care for Children.* Stein REK, ed. New York: United Hospital Fund of New York, 1997: 1–11.

[188] Schor EL, Abrams M, Shea K. Medicaid: Health Promotion and Disease Prevention for School Readiness. *Health Affairs* 26 (2007): 420–429; Pittard W, Laditka SB, Laditka JN, Xirasagar S, et al. Infant Health Outcomes Differ Notably among Medicaid Insurance Models: Evidence of a Successful Case Management Program in South Carolina. *J SC Med Assoc* 103 (2007): 228–233; Gavin NI, Adams EK, Hertz EJ, Chawla AJ, et al. The Use of EPSDT and Other Healthcare Services by Children Enrolled in Medicaid: The Impact of OBRA '89. *Milbank Quarterly* 76, no. 2 (1998): 207–232; Pittard WB, Laditka JN, Laditka SB. Associations between Early and Periodic Screening, Diagnosis, and Treatment and Health Outcomes among Medicaid Insured Infants in South Carolina. *J of Pediatrics* 151 (2007): 414–418; and Pittard, WB, Hulsey TC, Laditka JN, Laditka SB. School Readiness among Children Insured by Medicaid in South Carolina. *Prev Chronic Dis* 9 (2012) Available at: http://www.cdc.gov/pcd/issues/2012/11 0333.htm. Accessed: August 22, 2013.

[189] Committee on Practice and Ambulatory Medicine, Bright Futures Steering Committee. Recommendations for Preventive Pediatric Health Care. *Pediatrics* 120, no. 6 (2007): 1376. http://dx.doi.org/10.1542/peds.2007-2901; and Tanski S, Garfunkel LC, Duncan PM, Weitzman M. Performing Preventive Services: A Bright Futures Handbook. Available at: http://brightfutures.aap.org/continuing_education.html. Accessed May 5, 2012.

[190] Gavin et al. Use of EPSDT. 207–232.

[191] Tanski et al. Performing Preventive Services.

[192] Tanski et al. Performing Preventive Services; Ruff HA, Bijur PE, Markowitz M, Ma YC, Rosen JF. Declining Blood Lead Levels and Cognitive Changes in Moderately Lead-Poisoned Children. *JAMA* 269,

no. 13 (1993): 1641–1646; and Lozoff B. Iron and Learning Potential in Childhood. *Bulletin of the New York Academy of Medicine* 65, no. 10 (1989): 1050–1066.

[193] Schor et al. Medicaid: Health Promotion. 420–429; Dev LS, Shrivastava N. Anticipatory guidance. *Clin Fam Pract* 5, no. 2 (2003): 313–42. http://dx.doi.org/10.1016/S1522-5720(03)00028-X; Currie J. Health Disparities and Gaps in School Readiness. *Future Child.* 15, no.1 (2005): 117–138; Dworkin PH. Ready to Learn: A Mandate for Pediatrics. *J Dev Behav Pediatr* 14, no.3 (1993): 192–196; and Oja L, Jurimae T. Physical Activity, Motor Ability, and School Readiness of 6-year Old Children. *Percep Mot Skills* 95, no. 2 (2002): 407–15.

[194] Dev and Shrivastava. Anticipatory guidance. 313–42; and Weitzman M. The Role of the Individual Child Health Care Practitioner. *Health Care for Children*. Stein REK, ed. New York: United Hospital Fund of New York, 1997: 135–57.

[195] Ruff et al. Declining Blood Lead Levels. 1641–1646; and Burke H, Leonardi-Bee J, Hashim A, Pine-Abata H, et al. Prenatal and Passive Smoke Exposure and Incidence of Asthma and Wheeze: Systematic Review and Meta-analysis. *Pediatrics* 129, no. 4 (2012): 735–744.

[196] Tanski et al. Performing Preventive Services.

[197] Schor et al. Medicaid: Health Promotion. 420–429; Ruff et al. Declining Blood Lead Levels. 1641–1646; Currie. Health Disparities. 117–138; Dworkin. Ready to Learn. 192–196; Oja and Jurimae. Physical Activity. 407–15; Willis E, Kabler-Babbitt C, Zuckerman B. Early Literacy Interactions: Reach Out and Read. *Pediatr Clin North Am* 54, no. 3 (2007): 625–642. PubMed http://dx.doi.org/10.1016/j.pcl.2007.02.012; Lloyd JE, Li L, Hertzman C. Early Experiences Matter: Lasting Effect of Concentrated Disadvantage on Children's Language and Cognitive Outcomes. *Health Place* 16, no. 2 (2010): 371–380. PubMed. http://dx.doi.org/10.1016/j.healthplace.2009.11.009; Raikes H, Pan BA, Luze G, Tamis-LeMonda CS, Brooks-Gunn J, Constantine L, et al. Mother-Child Bookreading in Low-Income Families: Correlates and Outcomes During the First Three Years of Life. *Child Dev* 77, no. 4 (2006): 924–953. PubMed. http://dx.doi.org/10.1111/j.1467-8624.2006.00911.x; Magnuson KA, Waldfogel J. Early Childhood Care and Education: Effects on Ethnic and Racial Gaps in School Readiness. *Future Child* 15, no. 1 (2005): 169–196. PubMed. http://dx.doi.org/10.1353/foc.2005.0005; and Aber JL, Bennett NG, Conley DC, Li J. The Effects of Poverty on Child Health and Development. *Annu Rev Public Health* 18 (1997): 463–483. PubMed. http://dx.doi.org/10.1146/annurev.publhealth.18.1.463.

[198] Schor EL. Rethinking Well-Child Care. *Pediatrics* 114, no. 1 (2004): 210–216.

[199] Grason H, Morreale M. Health Services for Children and Adolescents: A "Non-System" of Care. *Health Care for Children: What's Right, What's*

Wrong, and What's Next. Stein REK and Brookes P, eds. New York: United Hospital Fund, 1997; and Farel AM and Kotch JB. The Child from One to Four: The Toddler and Preschool Years. *Maternal and Child Health: Programs, Problems, and Policy in Public Health.* Kotch JB, ed. Gaithersburg, MD: Aspen Publications, 1997.

[200] Grason and Morreale. Health Services; and Gavin et al. Use of EPSDT. 207–232.

[201] Hakim RB, Bye BV. Effectiveness of Compliance with Pediatric Preventive Care Guidelines among Medicaid Beneficiaries. *Pediatrics* 108, no. 1 (2001): 90–97.

[202] Wood DL, Hayward RA, Corey CR, et al. Access to Medical Care for Children and Adolescents in the United States. *Pediatrics* 86 (1990): 666–673; and Fox, H. An Examination of State Medicaid Financing Arrangements of Early Childhood Development Services. *Maternal and Child Health Journal* 4 (2000): 19–27.

[203] Pittard et al. Infant Health Outcomes. 228–233; Pittard et al. Associations between Early and Periodic. 414–418; Pittard et al. School Readiness; Pittard WB. Well Child Care in Infancy and Emergency Department Use by South Carolina Medicaid Children Birth to Six Years. *Southern Medical Journal* 104, no. 8 (2011): 604–608; and Peterson LA, Burstin HR, O'Neil AC, Orav EJ, et al. Non-Urgent Emergency Department Visits: The Effect of Having a Regular Doctor. *Medical Care* 36 (1998): 1249–1255.

[204] Hakim and Bye. Effectiveness of Compliance. 90–97.

[205] American Academy of Pediatrics. Recommendations for Preventive Health Care of Children and Youth. News and Comments. *American Academy of Pediatrics* 25, no. 6 (1974).

[206] Pittard et al. Associations between Early and Periodic. 414–418; Pittard et al. School Readiness; Pittard. Well Child Care. 604–608; and Shadish WR, Cook TD, Campbell DT. *Experimental and Quasi-Experimental Design for Generalized Causal Inference.* New York: Houghton Mifflin Company, 2002.

[207] US Congress, Office of Technology Assessment, Healthy Children: Investing in the Future, chapter 6, pages 119–144, OTA-H-345. Washington, DC: US Government Printing Office, February 1988.

[208] Shadish et al. *Experimental and Quasi-Experimental.*

[209] Ibid.

[210] Pittard et al. Associations between Early and Periodic. 414–418; Pittard et al. School Readiness; and Pittard. Well Child Care. 604–608.

[211] Pittard et al. Associations between Early and Periodic. 414–418; and Pittard et al. School Readiness.

[212] Weitzman. Role of the Individual. 135–57; and US Congress, Office of Technology Assessment. 119–144.

[213] Schor. Rethinking Well-Child Care. 210–216.

[214] Chassin MR, Galvin RW, and the National Roundtable on Health Care Quality. The Urgent Need to Improve Health Care Quality. *Journal of the American Medical Association* 280 (1998): 1000–1005.

[215] Russell BL. *Is Prevention Better Than Cure?* Washington, DC: The Brookings Institution: 1986.

[216] Weitzman. Role of the Individual. 135–57; US Congress, Office of Technology Assessment. 119–144; and Anastasi A. *Psychological Testing.* New York: Macmillan, 1988.

[217] Pittard et al. Associations between Early and Periodic. 414–418; Pittard et al. School Readiness; Pittard. Well Child Care. 604–608; and Anastasi, *Psychological Testing.*

[218] Schor. Rethinking Well-Child Care. 210–216; and Radecki L, Olson LM, Frintner MP, Tanner JL, et al. What Do Families Want from Well-Child Care? Including Parents in the Rethinking Discussion. *Pediatrics* 124, no. 3 (2008): 858–865.

[219] US Congress, Office of Technology Assessment. 119–144.

[220] Schor. Rethinking Well-Child Care. 210–216.

[221] Schor. Rethinking Well-Child Care. 210–216; US Congress, Office of Technology Assessment. 119–144; and Telfair J, Kotch JB. The School Age Child from Five to Nine. *Maternal and Child Health.* Kotch JB, ed. Gaithersburg, Maryland: Aspen Publishers, Inc., 1997: 147–171.

[222] The Politics of Evidence-Based Medicine. An Agency for Healthcare Research and Quality Available at: http://www.ahrq.gov/clinic/jhppl/rodwin.htm. Accessed: August 18, 2013; and Moyer VA, Butler M. Gaps in the Evidence for Well-Child Care: A Challenge to Our Profession. *Pediatrics* 114, no. 6 (2004): 1511–1521.

[223] Newman DH. Believing in Treatments That Don't Work. Available at: http://well.blogs.nytimes.com/2009/04/02/the-ideology-of-health-care. Accessed: May 11, 2012.

[224] Moyer and Butler. Gaps in the Evidence. 1511–1521; and Hoekelman RA. An Appraisal of the Effectiveness of Child Health Supervision. *Curr Opin Pediatr* 1 (1989): 146–155.

[225] Schor et al. Medicaid: Health Promotion. 420–429; and Schor. Rethinking Well-Child Care. 210–216.

[226] Moyer and Butler. Gaps in the Evidence. 1511–1521; and Weitzman. M. The Role of the Individual Child Health Care Practitioner. *Health Care for Children: What's Right, What's Wrong, and What's Next.* Stein REK and Brookes P, eds. 1997. New York: United Hospital Fund.

[227] Shadish et al. *Experimental and Quasi-Experimental.*

[228] Pittard et al. Associations between Early and Periodic. 414–418; Pittard et al. School Readiness; and Pittard. Well Child Care. 604–608.

[229] Pittard et al. Associations between Early and Periodic. 414–418.

[230] Alexander GR, Himes JH, Kaufman RB, Mor J, et al. A United States National Reference for Fetal Growth. *Obstet Gynecol* 87, no. 2 (1996): 163–168; and Hamilton BE, Martin JA, Sutton PD. Births: Preliminary Data for 2003. *Natl Vital Stat Rep* 53 (2004): 1–17.

[231] Falik M, Needleman J, Wells BL, Korb J. Ambulatory Care Sensitive Hospitalization and Emergency Visits: Experiences of Medicaid Patients Using Federally Qualified Health Centers. *Med Care* 39 (2001): 551–561.

[232] Pittard. Well Child Care. 604–608.

[233] Schor et al. Medicaid: Health Promotion. 420–429; Gavin et al. Use of EPSDT. 207–232; Pittard et al. School Readiness; Schor. Rethinking Well-Child Care. 210–216; Wold C, Nicholas W. Starting to School Healthy and Ready to Learn: Using Social Indicators to Improve School Readiness in Los Angeles County. *Preventing Chronic Disease* 4 (2007): A106; and Byrd R, Hoekelman R, Auinger P. Adherence to AAP Guidelines for Well-Child Care Under Managed Care. *Pediatrics* 104 (1999): 536–540.

[234] Dev and Shrivastava. Anticipatory guidance. 313–42; and Aber et al. Effects of Poverty. 463–483.

[235] Willis et al. Early Literacy Interactions. 625–642; and Wold and Nicholas. Starting to School. A106.

[236] Schor et al. Medicaid: Health Promotion. 420–429.

[237] Pittard et al. School Readiness.

[238] Ruff et al. Declining Blood Lead Levels. 1641–1646; Lozoff. Iron and Learning Potential. 1050–1066; Dev and Shrivastava. Anticipatory guidance. 313–42; Dworkin. Ready to Learn. 192–196; Lloyd. Early Experiences Matter. 371–380; and Lunkenheimer ES, Dishion TJ, Shaw DS, Connell AM, et al. Collateral Benefits of the Family Check-Up on Early Childhood School Readiness: Indirect Effects of Parents' Positive Behavior Support. *Dev Psychol* 44, no. 6 (2008): 1737–1752. PubMed. http://dx.doi.org/10.1037/a0013858.

[239] Schor et al. Medicaid: Health Promotion. 420–429; Currie. Health Disparities. 117–138; Raikes et al. Mother-Child Bookreading. 924–953; and Zuckerman B, Stevens G, Inkelas M, Halfon M. Prevalence and Correlates of High Quality Basic Pediatric Preventive Care. *Pediatrics* 114 (2004): 1522–1529.

[240] Schor et al. Medicaid: Health Promotion. 420–429; Ruff et al. Declining Blood Lead Levels. 1641–1646; Oja and Jurimae. Physical Activity. 407–15; Willis et al. Early Literacy Interactions. 625–642; and Raikes et al. Mother-Child Bookreading. 924–953.

[241] Pittard et al. School Readiness; and Pittard. Well Child Care. 604–608.

[242] Farel and Kotch. Child from One to Four; and Pittard. Well Child Care. 604–608

[243] Schor et al. Medicaid: Health Promotion. 420–429; Pittard et al. School Readiness; Pittard. Well Child Care. 604–608; and Grason and Morreale. Health Services for Children.

[244] Pittard et al. School Readiness; and Pittard. Well Child Care. 604–608.

[245] Pittard. Well Child Care. 604–608.

[246] Pittard et al. School Readiness.

[247] Chassin et al. Urgent Need to Improve. 1000–1005; and Russell. *Is Prevention Better?*

[248] Plotkin SA, Plotkin SL. A Short History of Vaccination. *Vaccines,* fifth edition. Plotkin SA, Orenstein WA, Offit PA, eds. Philadelphia: Saunders/Elsevier, 2013: 1–13.

[249] Offit PA. Vaccine Education Center. History of the Vaccine Schedule, 2012. http://www.chop.edu/service/vaccine-education-center/vaccine-schedule/history-of-vaccine-schedule.html. Accessed April 1, 2013, 2013; and Centers for Disease Control and Prevention. Immunization Schedules. Past Immunization Schedules, 2013. http://www.cdc.gov/vaccines/schedules/past.html. Accessed: March 30, 2013, 2013.

[250] Plotkin and Plotkin. Short History of Vaccination. 1–13.

[251] Smith PJ, Wood D, Darden PM. Highlights of Historical Events Leading to National Surveillance of Vaccination Coverage in the United States. *Public Health Rep* 126, Suppl 2 (July–August 2011): 3–12; and Aronson SM, Newman L. Smallpox in the Americas 1492 to 1815: Contagion and Controversy. 2002. http://www.brown.edu/Administration/News_Bureau/2002-03/02-017t.html. Accessed: April 1, 2013.

[252] Smith et al. Highlights of Historical Events. 3–12; and Bernstein SS. Smallpox and Variolation: Their Historical Significance in the American Colonies. *Journal of the Mount Sinai Hospital, New York* 18, no. 4 (November–December 1951): 228–244.

[253] Jackson CL. State Laws on Compulsory Immunization in the United States. *Public Health Rep* 84, no. 9 (September 1969): 787–795.

[254] Robbins KB, Brandling-Bennett D, Hinman AR. Low Measles Incidence: Association with Enforcement of School Immunization Laws. *American Journal of Public Health* 71, no. 3 (March 1981): 270–274; Orenstein WA, Halsey NA, Hayden GF, et al. From the Center for Disease Control: Current Status of Measles in the United States, 1973–1977. *The Journal of Infectious Diseases* 137, no. 6 (June 1978): 847–853; and Orenstein WA, Hinman AR. The Immunization System in the United States—The Role of School Immunization Laws. *Vaccine* 17 Suppl 3 (October 29 1999): S19–24.

[255] Salmon DA, Sapsin JW, Teret S, et al. Public Health and the Politics of School Immunization Requirements. *American Journal of Public Health* 95, no. 5 (May 2005): 778–783.

[256] Centers for Disease Control and Prevention. Recommended Childhood Immunization Schedule—United States, January 1995. Advisory Committee on Immunization Practices. American Academy of Pediatrics. American Academy of Family Physicians. National Immunization Program, CDC. *Morb Mortal Wkly Rep* 43, no. 51–52 (January 6, 1995): 959–960; and Smith JC, Snider DE, Pickering LK, Advisory Committee on Immunization P. Immunization Policy Development in the United States: The Role of the Advisory Committee on Immunization Practices. *Annals of Internal Medicine* 150, no. 1 (January 6, 2009): 45–49.

[257] Offit PA. History of the Vaccine Schedule.

[258] Henderson DA. Smallpox Eradication. *Public Health Rep* 95, no. 5 (September–October 1980): 422–426.

[259] Centers for Disease Control. Immunization Schedules; and Immunization Practices Advisory Committee, Centers for Disease Control. General Recommendations on Immunization. Recommendation of the Immunization Practices Advisory Committee. *Annals of Internal Medicine* 98, no. 5 pt 1 (May 1983): 615–622.

[260] Centers for Disease. Recommended Childhood Immunization. 959–960; and Hall CB. The Recommended Childhood Immunization Schedule of the United States. Committee on Infectious Diseases, American Academy of Pediatrics and Center for Disease Control. *Pediatrics* 95, no. 1 (January 1995): 135–137.

[261] Centers for Disease Control and Prevention. Recommended Childhood and Adolescent Immunization Schedule—United States, 2006. *Morb Mortal Wkly Rep* 53, no. 51–52 (January 6, 2006): Q1–4. American Academy of Pediatrics. Recommended Childhood and Adolescent Immunization Schedule—United States, 2006. *Pediatrics* 117, no. 1 (January 2006): 239–240.

[262] Murphy TV, Gargiullo PM, Massoudi MS, et al. Intussusception among Infants Given an Oral Rotavirus Vaccine. *New England Journal of Medicine* 344, no. 8 (February 2001): 564–572; Centers for Disease Control and P. Rotavirus Vaccine for the Prevention of Rotavirus Gastroenteritis among Children. Recommendations of the Advisory Committee on Immunization Practices (ACIP). *Morb. Mortal. Wkly. Rep* 48, no. RR-2 (March 9, 1999): 1–20; Centers for Disease Control and P. Intussusception among Recipients of Rotavirus Vaccine—United States, 1998–1999. *Morb. Mortal. Wkly. Rep.* 48, no. 27 (July 16, 1999): 577–581; and Centers for Disease Control and P. Withdrawal of Rotavirus Vaccine Recommendation. *Morb. Mortal. Wkly. Rep.* 48, no. 43 (November 15, 1999): 1007.

[263] Pediatrics AAo, Committee on Infectious Diseases. Recommended Childhood and Adolescent Immunization Schedule—United States, 2013. *Pediatrics* 131, no. 2 (February 1, 2013): 397–398; and Centers for Disease Control and Prevention. Advisory Committee on Immunization Practices (ACIP) Recommended Immunization Schedules for Persons aged 0 through 18 Years—United States, 2013. *MMWR Surveill Summ* 62, Suppl 1 (February 1, 2013): 2–8.

[264] Collins SD. Frequency of Immunizing Procedures of Various Kinds in 9,000 Families Observed for 12 Months, 1928–1931. *Am J Public Health Nations Health* 25, no. 11 (November 1935): 1221–1225.

[265] Sirken MG, Brenner B. Population Characteristics and Participation in the Poliomyelitis Vaccination Program. *Public Health Monograph* 61 (1960): 1–37; and Simpson DM, Ezzati-Rice TM, Zell ER. Forty Years and Four Surveys: How Does Our Measuring Measure Up? *American Journal of Preventive Medicine* 20, no. 4 Suppl (May 2001): 6–14.

[266] Simpson et al. Forty Years. 6–14.

[267] Ibid.

[268] Jain N, Singleton JA, Montgomery M, Skalland B. Determining Accurate Vaccination Coverage Rates for Adolescents: The National Immunization Survey—Teen 2006. *Public Health Rep* 124, no. 5 (September–October 2009): 642–651; Smith PJ, Battaglia MP, Huggins VJ, et al. Overview of the Sampling Design and Statistical Methods Used in the National Immunization Survey. *American Journal of Preventive Medicine* 20, no. 4 Suppl (May 2001): 17–24; and Smith PJ, Hoaglin DC, Battaglia MP, Khare M, Barker LE. Statistical Methodology of the National Immunization Survey, 1994–2002. *Vital and Health Statistics* 138 (March 2005): 1–55.

[269] US Department of Health and Human Services. HealthyPeople 2020. 2010. www.healthypeople.gov/2020. Accessed: April 1, 2013.

[270] Ibid.

[271] Ibid.

[272] Ibid.

[273] Santibanez TA, Shefer A, Briere EC, Cohn AC, Groom AV. Effects of a Nationwide Hib Vaccine Shortage on Vaccination Coverage in the United States. *Vaccine* 30, no. 5 (January 20, 2012): 941–947; and Centers for Disease C, Prevention. Continued Shortage of Haemophilus Influenzae Type b (Hib) Conjugate Vaccines and Potential Implications for Hib Surveillance—United States, 2008. *Morb Mortal Wkly Rep* 57, no. 46 (November 21, 2008): 1252–1255.

[274] US Department of Health. HealthyPeople 2020.

[275] Collins. Frequency of Immunizing. 1221–1225.

[276] Marin M, Broder KR, Temte JL, et al. Use of Combination Measles, Mumps, Rubella, and Varicella Vaccine: Recommendations of the

Advisory Committee on Immunization Practices (ACIP). *MMWR Recomm Rep.* 59, no. RR-3 (May 7, 2010): 1–12.

[277] Orenstein and Hinman. Immunization System. S19–24.

[278] Centers for Disease. Continued Shortage. 1252–1255.

[279] Centers for Disease. Recommended Childhood Immunization. 959–960.

[280] Marin et al. Use of Combination Measles. 1–12.

[281] Centers for Disease. Intussusception among Recipients. 577–581.

[282] Centers for Disease. Advisory Committee on Immunization. 2–8.

[283] Meissner HC, Reef SE, Cochi S. Elimination of Rubella from the United States: A Milestone on the Road to Global Elimination. *Pediatrics* 117, no. 3 (March 2006): 933–935.

[284] Centers for Disease. Impact of Vaccines. 243–248.

[285] Rodewald LE, Orenstein WA, Hinman AR, Schuchat A. Immunization in the United States. *Vaccines,* fifth edition. Plotkin SA, Orenstein WA, Offit PA, eds. Philadelphia: Saunders/Elsevier; 2013: 1310–1333.

[286] Murphy et al. Intussusception among Infants. 564–572.

[287] Marin et al. Use of Combination Measles. 1–12.

[288] Santibanez et al. Effects of a Nationwide Hib Vaccine. 941–947.

[289] Cherry JD. Epidemic Pertussis in 2012—The Resurgence of a Vaccine-preventable Disease. *N Engl J Med* 367, no. 9 (August 30, 2012): 785–787.

[290] Centers for Disease Control and P. Update: Eradication of Paralytic Poliomyelitis in the Americas. *Morb. Mortal. Wkly. Rep.* 41, no. 36 (September 11, 1992): 681–683.

[291] Henderson. Smallpox Eradication. 422–426; and Rotz LD, Dotson DA, Damon IK, Becher JA, Advisory Committee on Immunization P. Vaccinia (smallpox) Vaccine: Recommendations of the Advisory Committee on Immunization Practices (ACIP), 2001. *MMWR Recomm Rep* 50, no. RR-10 (January 22, 2001): 1–25; quiz CE21–27.

[292] Katz SL, Hinman AR. Summary and Conclusions: Measles Elimination Meeting, 16–17 March 2000. *The Journal of Infectious Diseases* 189 Suppl 1 (May 1, 2004): S43–47.

[293] Meissner et al. Elimination of Rubella. 933–935.

[294] Centers for Disease Control and Prevention. Summary of Notifiable Diseases—United States, 2010. *Morb Mortal Wkly Rep* 59, no. 53 (June 1 2012): 1–111; Roush SW, Murphy TV, Vaccine-Preventable Disease Table Working Group. Historical Comparisons of Morbidity and Mortality for Vaccine-Preventable Diseases in the United States. *JAMA* 298, no. 18 (2007): 2155–2163; and Rodewald et al. Immunization in the United States. 1310–1333.

[295] Poehling KA, Szilagyi PG, Grijalva CG, et al. Reduction of Frequent Otitis Media and Pressure-equalizing Tube Insertions in Children

after Introduction of Pneumococcal Conjugate Vaccine. *Pediatrics* 119, no. 4 (April 2007): 707–715; Grijalva CG, Poehling KA, Nuorti JP, et al. National Impact of Universal Childhood Immunization with Pneumococcal Conjugate Vaccine on Outpatient Medical Care Visits in the United States. *Pediatrics* 118, no. 3 (September 2006): 865–873; Grijalva CG, Nuorti JP, Arbogast PG, Martin SW, Edwards KM, Griffin MR. Decline in Pneumonia Admissions after Routine Childhood Immunisation with Pneumococcal Conjugate Vaccine in the USA: A Time-series Analysis. *Lancet* 369, no. 9568 (April 7, 2007): 1179–1186; and Tsai CJ, Griffin MR, Nuorti JP, Grijalva CG. Changing Epidemiology of Pneumococcal Meningitis after the Introduction of Pneumococcal Conjugate Vaccine in the United States. *Clin Infect Dis* 46, no. 11 (June 1, 2008): 1664–1672.

[296] Lopez AS, Zhang J, Brown C, Bialek S. Varicella-related Hospitalizations in the United States, 2000–2006: The 1-dose Varicella Vaccination Era. *Pediatrics* 127, no. 2 (February 2011): 238–245.

[297] Zhou F, Shefer A, Weinbaum C, McCauley M, Kong Y. Impact of Hepatitis A Vaccination on Health Care Utilization in the United States, 1996–2004. *Vaccine* 25, no. 18 (May 4, 2007): 3581–3587.

[298] Cortes JE, Curns AT, Tate JE, et al. Rotavirus Vaccine and Health Care Utilization for Diarrhea in US Children. *N Engl J Med* 365, no. 12 (September 22, 2011): 1108–1117.

[299] Curns AT, Panozzo CA, Tate JE, et al. Remarkable Postvaccination Spatiotemporal Changes in United States Rotavirus Activity. *The Pediatric Infectious Disease Journal* 30, no. 1 Suppl (January 2011): S54–55.

[300] Tate JE, Haynes A, Payne DC, et al. Trends in National Rotavirus Activity before and after Introduction of Rotavirus Vaccine into the National Immunization Program in the United States, 2000–2012. *The Pediatric Infectious Disease Journal,* February 19, 2013.

[301] Katz and Hinman. Summary and Conclusions. S43–47.

[302] Cherry. Epidemic Pertussis. 785–787; Centers for Disease. Summary of Notifiable Diseases. 1–111; and Centers for Disease C, Prevention. Pertussis Epidemic—Washington, 2012. *Morb Mortal Wkly Rep* 61, no. 28 (July 20, 2012): 517–522.

[303] Zhou F, Santoli J, Messonnier ML, et al. Economic Evaluation of the 7-vaccine Routine Childhood Immunization Schedule in the United States, 2001. *Arch Pediatr Adolesc Med* 159, no. 12 (December 2005): 1136–1144.

[304] Maciosek MV, Edwards NM, Coffield AB, et al. Priorities among Effective Clinical Preventive Services: Methods. *American Journal of Preventive Medicine* 31, no. 1 (July 2006): 90–96.

[305] Maciosek MV, Coffield AB, Edwards NM, Flottemesch TJ, Goodman MJ, Solberg LI. Priorities among Effective Clinical Preventive Services: Results of a Systematic Review and Analysis. *American Journal of Preventive Medicine* 31, no. 1 (July 2006): 52–61.

[306] Rodewald et al. Immunization in the United States. 1310–1333; and Zhou et al. Economic Evaluation. 1136–1144.

[307] Centers for Disease. Impact of Vaccines. 243–248; and Centers for Disease. Ten Great Public Health. 241–243.

[308] Centers for Disease. Immunization Schedules.

[309] Centers for Disease. Recommended Childhood Immunization. 959–960.

[310] Centers for Disease. Recommended Childhood and Adolescent. Q1–4.

[311] Centers for Disease. Advisory Committee. 2–8.

[312] Rodewald et al. Immunization in the United States. 1310–1333.

[313] Centers for Disease. Summary of Notifiable Diseases. 1–111.

[314] Ibid.

[315] Committee on Practice and Ambulatory Medicine, Bright Futures Steering Committee. Recommendations for Preventive Pediatric Health Care. *Pediatrics* 120, no. 6 (2007): 1376. http://dx.doi.org/10.1542/peds.2007-2901.

[316] Ebbeling CB, Pawlak DB, Ludwig DS. Childhood Obesity: Public Health Crisis, Common Sense Cure. *Lancet* 360 (2002): 473–482. Available at: http://www.allhealth.org/briefingmaterials/lancetobesityrev-393-pdf. Accessed February 23, 2013; and Schor EL. Rethinking Well-Child Care. *Pediatrics* 114, no. 1 (2004): 210–216.

[317] Schor. Rethinking Well-Child Care. 210–216.

[318] CMS-1590-P-Revisions to Payment Policies Under the Physician Fee Schedule, DME Face-to-Face Encounters, Elimination of the Requirement for Termination of Non-Random Prepayment Complex Medical Review and Other Revisions to Part B for CY 2013. Available at: http://www.cms.gov/Medicare/Medicare-Fee-For-Service-Payment/PhysicianFeeSchedule/PFS-Federal-Regulations-Notices-Items/CNS-1590-P.html. Accessed: June 10, 2013.

[319] Department of Health and Human Services, Center for Medicare and Medicaid Services. Screening and Behavioral Counseling Interventions in Primary Care to Reduce Alcohol Misuse. Available at: http://www.cms.gov/Outreach-and-Education/Medicare-Learning-Network-MLN/MLNMattersArticles/downloads/MM7791.pdf. Accessed: February 20, 2013.

[320] Walker DM. Fiscal and Health Care Challenges. September 2007. Available at: http://www.gao.gov/cghome.htm. Accessed: March 6, 2013.

[321] Affordable Care Act. Available at: http://www.medicaid.gov/AffordableCareAct/Affordable-Care-Act.html. Accessed: March 5, 2013.

[322] American Academy of Pediatrics, Periodic Survey of Fellows 46. Elk Grove Village, IL: American Academy of Pediatrics, 2001.

[323] Peterson LA, Burstin HR, O'Neil AC, Orav EJ, et al. Non-Urgent Emergency Department Visits: The Effect of Having a Regular Doctor. *Medical Care* 36 (1998): 1249–1255.

[324] American Academy of Pediatrics. Periodic Survey.

[325] American Hospital Association Resource Center Blog. What's the Average Cost for an ER Visit? Posted July 27, 2011. Available at: http://www.meps.ahrq.gov/mpsweb/data_files/publications/st318/stat318.pdf. Accessed: March 3, 2013.

[326] Schor. Rethinking Well-Child Care. 210–216; and Hakim RB, Bye BV. Effectiveness of Compliance with Pediatric Preventive Care Guidelines among Medicaid Beneficiaries. *Pediatrics* 108, no. 1 (2001): 90–97.

[327] Margolis LH, Cole GP, Kotch JB. Historical Foundations of Maternal and Child Health. *Maternal and Child Health: Programs, Problems, and Policy in Public Health*. JB Kotch, ed. Gaithersburg, MD: Aspen Publications, 1997.

[328] American Academy of Pediatrics. Recommendations for Preventive Health Care of Children and Youth. News and Comments. Evanston, IL. *American Academy of Pediatrics* 25, no. 6 (1974).

[329] Inglehart J. Medicaid. *New Eng J Med* 340 (1999): 403–408.

[330] Health Resources and Services Administration. EPSDT Program Background. Available at: http://mchb.hrsa.gov/epsdt/overview.html. Accessed: March 14, 2013.

[331] Ibid.

[332] Early and Periodic Screening, Diagnosis, and Treatment Available at: http://www.medicaid.gov/Medicaid-CHIP-Program-Information/By-Topics/Benefits/Early-Periodic-Screening. Accessed: August 18, 2013; and Gavin NI, Adams EK, Hertz EJ, Chawla AJ, et al. The Use of EPSDT and Other Healthcare Services by Children Enrolled in Medicaid: The Impact of OBRA '89. *Milbank Quarterly* 76, no. 2 (1998): 207–232.

[333] Sardell A, Johnson K. The Politics of EPSDT Policy in the 1990s: Policy Entrepreneurs, Political Streams, and Children's Health Benefits. *Millbank Quarterly* 76 (1998): 175–205; and Sardell, A. The Paradox of Consensus. *J Health Policy, Politics, and Law* 15, no. 2 (1990): 271–304.

[334] Rosenbaum S, Johnson K, Sonosky C, Markus A, DeGraw C. The Children's Hour: The State Children's Health Insurance Program. *Health Affairs* 17, no. 1 (1998): 75–89.

[335] Rosenbaum, S. Medicaid. *New England Journal of Medicine* 346 (2002): 635–640; and Silberman P, Wettach JR. eds. *Health Insurance and Health Programs*. Raleigh, North Carolina: Publications Unlimited, 1995.

[336] Rosenbaum S, Johnson, K. Providing Health Care for Low-Income Children: Reconciling Child Health Goals with Child Health Financing Realities. *Millbank Quarterly* 64 (1986): 442–478.

[337] Monheit, A, Hogan, M, Berk, M, and Farley, P. The Employed Uninsured and the Role of Public Policy. Washington, DC, National Center for Health Services Research, 1984.

[338] Schlosberg, C, NHeLP, and Ferber, JD. Gateway Legal Services. Access to Medicaid Since the Personal Responsibility and Work Opportunity Reconciliation Act. 1998. Available at: http://www.healthlaw.org/pubs/med1998accessmedicaid.html. Accessed: March 22, 2013; and Perkins J and Schlosberg, C. National Health Law Program. The Welfare Law and Medicaid: Advocacy Tips for Making the Medicaid of the Savings Program Work. Available at: http://www.healthlaw.org/pubs/19961016welfare.html. Accessed: March 22, 2013.

[339] Center on Budget and Policy Priorities. Poverty Rate Fails to Decline as Income Growth in 1996 Favors the Affluent. 1997. Available at: www.cbpp.org/archiveSite/provday97.htm. Accessed: March 14, 2013.

[340] Rosenbaum et al. Children's Hour. 75–89.

[341] Sardell and Johnson. Politics of EPSDT. 175–205; and Ku L, Broaddus M, Wachino V. Medicaid and SCHIP Protected Insurance Coverage for Millions of Low Income Americans. Center on Budget and Policy Procedures, January 31, 2005. Available at: http://www.cbpp.org/cms/?fa=view&id=1013. Accessed: November 19, 2012.

[342] Child Trends Database. Healthcare Coverage. Available at: http://www.childtrendsdatabank.org/?q=node/116. Accessed: March 6, 2013.

[343] Centers for Medicare and Medicaid Services. The Deficit Reduction Act: Important Facts for State Government Officials. Available at: https://www.cms.gov/Regulations-and-Guidance/Legislation/Defic. Accessed: March 6, 2013.

[344] Muchmore S. Increase in Hospital Care Specialists Has Some Worried. Available at: http://www.tulsaworld.com/news/article.aspx?subjectid=17&articleid=20120508_17_A1_CUTLIN520644. Accessed: March 6, 2013.

[345] Pittard, WB, Laditka, SB, Laditka, JN, Xirasagar, S, and Lovelace, OF. Infant Health Outcomes Differ Notably among Medicaid Insurance Models: Evidence of a Successful Case Management Program in South Carolina. *Journal of the South Carolina Medical Association* 103 (2007): 188–193; and Pittard, WB, Laditka, JN, Xirasagar, S, and Laditka, SB. Infant Health Care Costs for Medicaid-Insured Infants in South Carolina

Enrolled in Three Insurance Plans from Birth to 24 Months. *Journal of the South Carolina Medical Association* 103 (2007): 194–197.

[346] Nielsen MN, Langner B, Zena C, Hacker T, Grundy P. Benefits of Implementing the Primary Care Patient-Centered Medical Home: A Review of Cost and Quality Results. Available at: http://www.pcpcc.net/files/benefits_of_implementing_the_primary_care_pcmh_0.pdf. Accessed: March 5, 2013.

[347] Muchmore. Increase in Hospital Care.

[348] Chasnoff IJ, Landress HJ, Barrett ME. The Prevalence of Illicit-Drug or Alcohol Use During Pregnancy and Discrepancies in Mandatory Reporting in Pinellas County, Florida. *N Engl J Med* 322 (1990): 1202–1206; and Duggan A, Windham A, McFarlane E, Fuddy L, Rohde C, Buchbinder S, Sia C. Hawaii's Healthy Start Program of Home Visiting for At-Risk Families: Evaluation of Family Identification, Family Engagement, and Service Delivery. *Pediatrics* 105, no. 1 (2000): 250–259.

[349] Early Experiences Matter: Love, Learning, and Routines. National Center for Infants, Toddlers, and Families. Available at: http://main.zerotothree.org/site/PageServer?pagename=ter_key_social_routines. Accessed: March 6, 2013; and Kuo AA, Franke TM, Regalado M, Halfon N. Parent Report of Reading to Young Children. *Pediatrics* 113 (2004): 1944–1951.

[350] Barnett, WS (1996). *Lives in the Balance: Benefit-cost Analysis of the Perry Preschool Program through Age 27.* Monographs of the High/Scope Educational Research Foundation. Ypsilanti, MI: High/Scope Press.

[351] Demerath EW, Schubert CM, Maynard M, Sun SS, Chumlea WC, Pickoff A, Czerwinski SA, Towne B, Siervogel RM. Do Changes in Body Mass Index Percentile Reflect Changes in Body Mass Composition in Children? Data from the Fels Longitudinal Study. *Pediatrics* 117, no. 3 (2006): e487–e495.

[352] Udall JN, Harrison GG, Vaucher Y, Walson PD, Morrow G. Interaction of Maternal and Neonatal Obesity. *Pediatrics* 62, no. 1 (1978): 17–21.

[353] US Health in International Perspective. The National Academy Press. 2013. Available at: www.nap.edu/catalog.php?record_id=13497. Accessed: March 6, 2013.

[354] Parker L, Burns AC, Sanchez E. Local Government Actions to Prevent Childhood Obesity. Institute of Medicine and National Research Council. Available at: http://www.nap.edu/catalog/12674.html. Accessed: March 6, 2013.

[355] The World Economic Forum and the Harvard School of Public Health. 2011. The Global Economic Burden of Non-Communicable Diseases. Available at: http://www3.weforum.org/WEF_Harvard

_HE_GlobalEconomicBurdenNonCommunicableDiseases. Accessed: March 6, 2013.

[356] Farel AM and Kotch JB. The Child from One to Four: The Toddler and Preschool Years. *Maternal and Child Health: Programs, Problems, and Policy in Public Health.* Kotch JB, ed. Gaithersburg, MD: Aspen Publications, 1997; and Starfield B. Social, Economic, and Medical Care Determinants of Children's Health. *Health Care for Children: What's Right, What's Wrong, and What's Next.* Stein REK and Brookes P, eds. New York: United Hospital Fund.

[357] US Health in International Perspective. National Academy Press.

[358] Ibid.

[359] Ortiz DD. Improving the Delivery of Preventive Services to Children. *American Family Physician* 83, no. 6 (2011): 659–666.

[360] Schor. Rethinking Well-Child Care. 210–216; Yankauer A, Lawrence RA. A Study of Periodic School Medical Examinations: Part II: The Annual Increment of New "Defects." *Am J Public Health* 46 (1956): 1553–1562; Sturner RA, Funk SG, Green JA. Simultaneous Technique for Acuity and Readiness Testing (START): Further Concurrent Validation of an Aid for Developmental Surveillance. *Pediatrics* 93 (1994): 82–88; Dworkin PH. British and American Recommendations for Developmental Monitoring: The Role of Surveillance. *Pediatrics* 84 (1989): 1000–1010; National Initiative for Children's Healthcare Quality. *A Practical Guide to Implementing Office Systems for Anticipatory Guidance.* Boston: National Initiative for Children's Healthcare Quality, 2002; Oehlmann P, Martin C. *Improving Preventive Care Services for Children Toolkit.* Lawrenceville, NJ: Center for Health Care Strategies. 2002; and Kilo CM, Triffletti P, Tantau C, Murray M. Improving Access to Clinical Offices. *J Med Pract Manage* 16 (2000): 126–132.

[361] Schor. Rethinking Well-Child Care. 210–216; and Ortiz. Improving the Delivery. 659–666.

[362] Schor. Rethinking Well-Child Care. 210–216; and American Academy of Pediatrics. Periodic Survey.

[363] Committee on Practice and Ambulatory Medicine: Bright Futures Steering Committee. Recommendations for Preventive Pediatric Health Care. *Pediatrics* 120 (2007): 1376; and Tanski S, Garfunkel LC, Duncan PM, Weitzman M. Performing Preventive Services: A Bright Futures Handbook. Available at: http://brightfutures.aap.org/continuing_education.html. Accessed: May 5, 2012.

[364] Tanski et al. Performing Preventive Services; Currie J. Health Disparities and Gaps in School Readiness. *The Future of Children* 15, no. 1 (2005): 117–138; Dworkin PH. Ready to Learn: A Mandate for Pediatrics. *J Dev Behav Pediatr* 14, no. 3 (1993): 192–96; Ruff HA, Bijur PE, Markowitz M, Yeou-Cheng M, Rosen JF. Declining Blood Lead Levels and Cognitive

Changes in Moderately Lead Poisoned Children. *JAMA* 269, no. 13 (1993): 1641–1646; Dev LS. Shrivastava N. Anticipatory Guidance. *Clinics in Family Practice* 5, no. 2 (2003): 313–341; and Oja L, Jurimae T. Physical Activity, Motor Ability, and School Readiness of 6-Year Old Children. *Percept Mot Skills* 95, no. 2 (2002): 407–415.

[365] Committee on Practice. Recommendations for Preventive Pediatric. 1376.

[366] Gavin NI, Adams EK, Hertz EI. The Use of EPSDT and Other Healthcare Services by Children Enrolled in Medicaid: The Impact of OBRA '89. *Milbank Quarterly* 76 (1998): 207–232.

[367] Committee on Practice. Recommendations for Preventive Pediatric. 1376; Dev and Shrivastava. Anticipatory Guidance. 313–341; Oja and Jurimae. Physical Activity. 407–415; Farel AM and Kotch JB. The Child from One to Four: The Toddler and Preschool Years. *Maternal and Child Health: Programs, Problems, and Policy in Public Health.* Kotch JB, ed. Gaithersburg, MD: Aspen Publications. 1997; and Charney E. Well-Child Care Axiom. *Well-Child Care. Report of the Seventeenth Ross Roundtable on Critical Approaches to Common Pediatric Problems.* Charney E, ed. Columbus, Ohio: Ross Laboratories, 1986.

[368] Starfield B and Shi L. The Medical Home, Access to Care, and Insurance: A Review of Evidence. *Pediatrics* 113, no. 6 (2004): 1493–1498; Byrd R, Hoekelman R, and Auinger P. Adherence to AAP Guidelines for Well-Child Care under Managed Care. *Pediatrics* 104 (1999): 536–540; Zuckerman B, Stevens G, Inkelas M, Halfon N. Prevalence and Correlates of High Quality Basic Pediatric Preventive Care. *Pediatrics* 114 (2004): 1522–1529; Telfair J and Kotch JB. The School-Age Child from Five to Nine. *Maternal and Child Health: Programs, Problems, and Policy in Public Health.* Kotch JB, ed. Gaithersburg, MD: Aspen Publications, 1997.

[369] Grason H, Morreale M. Health Services for Children and Adolescents: A "Non-System" of Care. *Health Care for Children: What's Right, What's Wrong, and What's Next.* Stein REK and Brookes P, eds. New York: United Hospital Fund. 1997.

[370] Hakim RB, Bye BV. Effectiveness of Compliance with Pediatric Preventive Care Guidelines among Medicaid Beneficiaries. *Pediatrics* 108 (2001): 90–97; Pittard, WB, Laditka, SB, Laditka, JN, Xirasagar, S, and Lovelace, OF. Infant Health Outcomes Differ Notably among Medicaid Insurance Models: Evidence of a Successful Case Management Program in South Carolina. *Journal of the South Carolina Medical Association* 103 (2007): 188–193; and Pittard, W, Laditka, J, and Laditka, S. Associations between Early and Periodic Screening, Diagnosis, and Treatment and Health Outcomes Among Medicaid Insured Infants in South Carolina. *J. Pediatrics* 151 (2007): 414–418.

[371] Pittard, William B. Well Child Care in Infancy and Emergency Department Use by South Carolina Medicaid Children Birth to Six Years Old. *Southern Medical Journal* 104, no. 8 (2011): 604–608.

[372] Zuckerman et al. Prevalence and Correlates. 1522–1529; and Telfair and Kotch. School-Age Child.

[373] Pittard WB, Hulsey TC, Laditka JN, Laditka SB. School Readiness Among Children Insured by Medicaid, in South Carolina. *Prev Chronic Dis.* 2012. Available at: http://www.cdc.gov//pcd/issues/2012/11 0333.htm. Accessed: August 22, 2013; and Russell BL. Is Prevention Better Than Cure? Washington, DC: The Brookings Institution, 1986.

[374] Committee on Practice. Recommendations for Preventive Pediatric. 1376.

[375] Ibid.; and Schor EL. Rethinking Well-Child Care. *Pediatrics* 114, no. 1 (2004): 210–216.

[376] Pittard et al. Infant Health Outcomes. 188–193; Pittard et al. Associations between Early and Periodic. 414–418; Pittard. Well Child Care. 604–608; and Pittard et al. School Readiness.

[377] Pittard et al. Infant Health Outcomes. 188–193.

[378] Pittard, WB, Laditka, JN, Xirasagar, S, and Laditka, SB. Infant Health Care Costs for Medicaid-Insured Infants in South Carolina Enrolled in Three Insurance Plans from Birth to 24 Months. *Journal of the South Carolina Medical Association* 103 (2007): 194–197; and Pittard, William B. Well Child Care in Infancy and Health Care Costs Birth–Six Years for South Carolina Medicaid Children. *Journal of the South Carolina Medical Association* 107, no. 10 (2011): 178–182.

[379] Rosenbaum, S. Medicaid. *New England Journal of Medicine* 346 (2002): 635–640; and Silberman P, Wettach JR. eds. Health Insurance and Health Programs. Raleigh, North Carolina. Publications Unlimited, 1995.

[380] DePark, N. A Profile of Medicaid, Chartbook 2000. United States Department of Health and Human Services; and Hurley R, Freund D, Paul J. Managed-Care in Medicaid. Ann Arbor, Michigan: Health Administration Press, 1993.

[381] Silberman and Wettach, eds. Health Insurance; and Medicare and Medicaid Programs: Change of Agency Name: Technical Amendments. A Rule by the Public Health Service, the Centers for Medicare and Medicaid Services, the Family Assistance Office, the Children and Families Administration, and the Child Support Enforcement Office on 7-31-2001. Available at: www.federalregister.gov/articles/2001/07/31/01-1859/medic. Accessed: November 28, 2012.

[382] Davis K, Schoen C. Health and the War on Poverty: A Ten-Year Appraisal. Washington, DC: Brookings Institution, 1978; and Rosenbaum S, Proser M, Sonosky C. Health Policy and Early Child Development: An

Overview. George Washington University: The Commonwealth Fund, June 2001.

[383] Gavin et al. Use of EPSDT. 207–232.

[384] Newacheck PW, Halfon N. Preventive Care Use by School-aged Children: Differences by Socioeconomic Status. *Pediatrics* 64 (1979): 304–309; Kasper JD. The Importance of Type of Usual Source of Care for Children's Physician Access and Expenditures. *Medical Care* 25 (1987): 386–398; Newacheck PW. Access to Ambulatory Care for Poor Persons. *Health Service Research* 23 (1988): 402–419; Rosenbach ML. The Impact of Medicaid on Physician Use by Low-Income Children. *American Journal of Public Health* 79 (1989): 220–226; Short PF, Lefkowitz DF. Encouraging Preventive Services for Low-Income Children: The Effect of Expanding Medicaid. *Medical Care* 30 (1992): 766–80; and Marquis MS, Long SH. Reconsidering the Effect of Medicaid on Healthcare Services Use. *Health Services* 30 (1996): 791–808.

[385] Wood DL, Hayward RA, Corey CR, et al. Access to Medical Care for Children and Adolescents in the United States. *Pediatrics* 86 (1990): 666–673; and Fox, H. An Examination of State Medicaid Financing Arrangements of Early Childhood Development Services. *Maternal and Child Health Journal* 4 (2000): 19–27.

[386] Sardell A, Johnson K. The Politics of EPSDT Policy in the 1990s: Policy Entrepreneurs, Political Streams, and Children's Health Benefits. *Milbank Quarterly* 76 (1998): 175–205; and Rosenbaum S, Johnson K. Providing Health Care for Low-Income Children: Reconciling Child Health Goals with Child Health Financing Realities. *Milbank Quarterly* 64 (1986): 442–478.

[387] Sardell and Johnson. Politics of EPSDT. 175–205; Rosenbaum and Johnson. Providing Health Care. 442–478; Butler, J, Winter W, Singer J. et al. Medical Care Use and Expenditures among US Children and Youth: Analysis of a National Probability Sample. *Pediatrics* 76 (1985): 495–503; Kleinman J. Use of Ambulatory Health Care by the Poor: Another Look at Equity. *Medical Care* 19 (1981): 1011–1019; and Rosenbaum S. The Prevention of Infant Mortality: The Unfulfilled Promise of Federal Health Programs for the Poor. *Clearinghouse Review* 17 (1983): 701–735.

[388] Sardell and Johnson. Politics of EPSDT. 175–205; and Sardell A. Child Health Policy in the US: The Paradox of Consensus. *The Health Policy and the Disadvantages*. LD Brown, ed. Durham, North Carolina: Duke University Press, 1991.

[389] Dubey L, Kenny G. Expanding Public Health Insurance to Parents: Effects on Children's Coverage Under Medicaid. *Health Services Research* 38 (2003): 1285–1301.

[390] Ku L, Broaddus M, Wachino V. Medicaid and SCHIP Protected Insurance Coverage for Millions of Low Income Americans. Center on Budget and Policy Procedures, January 31, 2005. Available at: http://www.cbpp.org/cms/?fa=view&id=1013. Accessed: November 19, 2012.

[391] Iglehart J. Medicaid. *New Engl J. Med* 340 (1999): 403–408.

[392] America's Children: Health Insurance and Access to Care. The National Academic Press. Available at: http://www.nap.edu/openbook.php?record_id=61688&p=87. Accessed: May 29, 2013.

[393] Iglehart J. Medicaid Turns to Prepaid Managed-Care. *N Engl J Med* 308 (1993): 976–980.

[394] Iglehart. Medicaid. 403–408; and Iglehart. Medicaid Turns to Prepaid. 976–980.

[395] Silberman and Wettach, eds. Health Insurance; Pittard WB. Our Expanding South Carolina Medicaid Managed Care Program. *Journal of the South Carolina Medical Association* 95 (1999): 9–13; and Pittard WB. Preventive Care Utilization by Medicaid Infants: Variation with South Carolina Health Care Models. *Journal of the South Carolina Medical Association* 100 (2004): 70–75.

[396] Kongstvedt P. The Managed Healthcare Handbook. Aspen Publishers Inc., Gaithersburg, Maryland, 1996.

[397] Silberman and Wettach, eds. Health Insurance.

[398] Comments from South Carolina DHHS Medicaid personnel, spring 2005.

[399] Chassin MR, Galvin RW. The Urgent Need to Improve Health Care Quality; Institute of Medicine National Roundtable on Health Care Quality. *JAMA* 280 (1998): 1000–1005.

[400] Peterson LA, Burstin HR, O'Neil AC, Orav EJ, et al. Non-Urgent Emergency Department Visits: The Effect of Having a Regular Doctor. *Medical Care* 36 (1998): 1249–1255; and Falik M, Needleman J, Wells BL, et al. Ambulatory Care Sensitive Hospitalizations and Emergency Visits: Experiences of Medicaid Patients Using Federally Qualified Health Centers. *Med Care* 39 (2001): 551–561.

[401] Pittard et all. Associations between Early and Periodic. 414–418; and Pittard. Well Child Care. 604–608.

[402] Ginzberg, E. and Ostow, M. Managed Care—A Look Back and a Look Ahead. *New England Journal of Medicine* 336 (1997): 1018–1020.

[403] Peterson et al. Non-Urgent Emergency. 1249–1255.

[404] Miller R, Luft H. Does Managed Care Lead to Better or Worse Quality of Care? *Health Affairs* Millwood. 6, no. 5 (1997): 7–25.

[405] Kassirer J. Managed-Care and the Morality of the Marketplace. *The New England Journal of Medicine* 333 (1997): 50–52.

406 Ginzberg and Ostow. Managed Care. 1018–1020; and Kassirer. Managed-Care. 50–52.
407 Charney. Well-Child Care Axiom; Casey PH, Bradley RH, Caldwell HM, et al. Developmental Intervention: A Pediatric Clinical Review. *J Pediatrics* 95 (1979): 1–9; Korsch BM. Issues in Evaluating Child Health Supervision. *J Pediatrics* 75 (1985): 942–951; Lewis C. What Is the Evidence? *Am. J. Dis. Child* 122 (1971): 469–474; Shadish WR. A Review and Critique of Controlled Studies of the Effectiveness of Preventive Child Health Care. *Health Policy Quarterly* 2 (1982): 24–52; and Yankauer A. Child Health Supervision—Is It Worth It? *Pediatrics* 52 (1973): 272–279.
408 Telfair and Kotch. School-Age Child; Hakim and Bye. Effectiveness of Compliance. 90–97; and US Congress, Office of Technology Assessment. Healthy Children. 119–144.
409 Farel and Kotch. Child from One to Four; US Congress, Office of Technology Assessment. Healthy Children. 119–144; Black DAK. Inequalities in Health: Report of a Research Working Group. London, England: Department of Health and Social Services, 1980; and Starfield B. Social, Economic, and Medical Care Determinants of Children's Health. *Health Care for Children: What's Right, What's Wrong, and What's Next.* Stein REK and Brookes P, eds. New York: United Hospital Fund, 1997.
410 Pittard. Well Child Care. 604–608; and Pittard et al. School Readiness.
411 Shadish WR, Cook TD, Campbell DT. *Experimental and Quasi-Experimental Design for Generalized Causal Inference*, New York: Houghton Mifflin Company, 2002.
412 US Congress, Office of Technology Assessment. Healthy Children. 119–144.
413 Hoekelman RA. What Constitutes Adequate Well-Child Care? *Pediatrics* 55 (1975): 313–326.
414 Gilbert IR, Feldman W, Siegel LS, Mills A, Dunnett C, Stoddard S. How Many Well Baby Visits Are Needed in the First Two Years of Life? *Can Med Assoc J* 130 (1984): 957–961.
415 Klein M, Roghmann K, Woodward K, Charney E. The Impact of the Rochester Neighborhood Health Center on Hospitalization of Children, 1968 to 1970. *Pediatrics* 51, no. 5: 833–839.
416 Casey PH, White JK. Effect of the Pediatrician on the Mother-Infant Relationship. *Pediatrics* 65 (1990): 815–820; Chamberlain RW, Szumowski BA. A Follow-up Study of Parent Education in Pediatric Office Practices: Impact at Age Two and a Half. *Am J Public Health* 70 (1980): 1180–1188; Cullen KI. A Six-Year Controlled Trial of Prevention of Children's Behavior Disorders. *J Pediatrics* 68 (1976): 662–666; and Gutelius MF, Kirsch AD, MacDonald S, et al. Controlled Study of the

Child's Health Supervision: Behavioral Results. *Pediatrics* 60 (1977): 294–304.

[417] Pittard. Well Child Care. 604–608; and Pittard et al. School Readiness.

[418] Hakim and Bye. Effectiveness of Compliance. 90–97.

[419] Pittard et al. Infant Health Outcomes. 188–193; Pittard et al. Associations between Early and Periodic. 414–418; Pittard. Well Child Care. 604–608; Pittard et al. School Readiness; Pittard et al. Infant Health Care Costs. 194–197; and Pittard. Well Child Care. 178–182.

[420] Pittard. Our Expanding South Carolina. 9–13; and Pittard. Preventive Care Utilization. 70–75.

[421] American Academy of Pediatrics. Recommendations for Preventive.

[422] Pittard et al. Infant Health Outcomes. 188–193; Pittard et al. Associations between Early and Periodic. 414–418; Pittard. Well Child Care. 604–608; and Pittard et al. School Readiness.

[423] Gavin et al. Use of EPSDT. 207–232; Pittard et al. School Readiness; Russell. Is Prevention Better?; and Schor. Rethinking Well-Child Care. 210–216.

[424] Pittard et al. Infant Health Outcomes. 188–193; and Kongstvedt. Managed Healthcare Handbook.

[425] Pittard et al. Infant Health Outcomes. 188–193; Pittard et al. Associations between Early and Periodic. 414–418; Pittard. Well Child Care. 604–608; and Pittard et al. School Readiness.

[426] Pittard. Well Child Care. 604–608.

[427] Falik et al. Ambulatory Care Sensitive Hospitalizations. 551–561.

[428] Peterson et al. Non-Urgent Emergency. 1249–1255.

[429] Pittard et al. Infant Health Outcomes. 188–193; Pittard et al. Associations between Early and Periodic. 414–418; Pittard. Well Child Care. 604–608.

[430] Pittard et al. School Readiness.

[431] US Congress, Office of Technology Assessment. Healthy Children. 119–144.

[432] Wold, C and Nicholas W. Starting to School Healthy and Ready to Learn: Using Social Indicators to Improve School Readiness in Los Angeles County. *Preventing Chronic Disease* 4 (2007): A106; and Crnic K. Reconsidering School Readiness: Conceptual and Applied Perspectives. *Early Education and Development* 5 (1994): 99–105.

[433] Willis E, Kabler-Babbitt C, Zuckerman, B. Early Literacy Interventions: Reach Out and Read. *Pediatric Clinics of North America* 54 (2007): 625–642; and Williamson, D. NC Kindergartners from Low Income Families Face Disadvantage in School Readiness. April 23, 2001. Available at: http://www.unc.edu/news/archives/apr01/maxwell042301.htm. Accessed: February 8, 2011.

[434] Currie. Health Disparities. 117–138; Lunkenheimer, ES, Dishion, TJ, Shaw, DS, Connell, AM, Gardner, F, Wilson, MN, Skuban EM. Collateral Benefits of the Family Check-Up on Early Childhood School Readiness: Indirect Effects of Parents' Positive Behavior Support. *Dev Psychol* 44, no. 6 (2008): 1737–52; Raikes H, Pan BA, Luze G, Tamis-LeMonda CS, Brooks-Gunn J, Constantine J, Tarullo LB, Raikes HA, Rodriguez ET. Mother-Child Bookreading in Low-Income Families: Correlates and Outcomes during the First Three Years of Life. *Child Dev* 77, no. 4 (2006): 924–53; and Schor, EL, Abrams, M, Shea, K. Medicaid: Health Promotion and Disease Prevention for School Readiness. *Health Affairs* 26 (2007): 420–429.

[435] Ruff et al. Declining Blood Lead Levels. 1641–1646; Oja and Jurimae. Physical Activity. 407–415; Raikes et al. Mother-Child Bookreading. 924–53; and Schor et al. Medicaid: Health Promotion. 420–429.

[436] Dev and Shrivastava. Anticipatory Guidance. 313–341; Wold and Nicholas. Starting to School Healthy. A106; and Schor et al. Medicaid: Health Promotion. 420–429.

[437] Pittard et al. Infant Health Care. 194–197; and Pittard. Well Child Care. 178–182.

[438] Chassin and Galvin. Urgent Need to Improve. 1000–1005.

[439] Pittard et al. Infant Health Outcomes. 188–193; and Pittard et al. Infant Health Care. 194–197.

[440] Pittard. Well Child Care. 178–182.

[441] Chassin and Galvin. Urgent Need to Improve. 1000–1005.

[442] Pittard. Well Child Care. 604–608.

[443] Pittard. Well Child Care. 178–182.

[444] Chassin and Galvin. Urgent Need to Improve. 1000–1005.

[445] Preamble to the Constitution of the World Health Organization as Adopted by the International Health Conference, New York, 19–22 June 1946 by the Representatives of 61 States (Official Records of the World Health Organization, no. 2, p. 100) and Entered into Force on 7 April 1948.

[446] Pittard. Well Child Care. 604–608; and Pittard et al. School Readiness.

Index

f denotes figure; *t* denotes table

A

AAFP (American Academy of Family Practice)
   on continuity of care, 13, 18
   on immunization schedule, 69
AAP (American Academy of Pediatrics). *See* American Academy of Pediatrics (AAP)
ABR (auditory brainstem response), 28
acellular pertussis vaccine, 70, 74, 77
acid-fast bacilli (AFB), 43
ADDM (Autism and Developmental Disabilities Monitoring) (CDC), 36
ADHD (attention-deficit/hyperactivity disorder), 58, 86
Advisory Committee on Immunization Practices (ACIP) (AAP), 69, 78
Affordable Care Act, 87, 95
Aid to Families with Dependent Children (AFDC), 9, 89, 90, 101–102
amblyopia, 30, 31, 32
ambulatory care sensitive condition (ACSC) diagnoses/conditions, 2–3, 21, 55, 56, 62, 63, 65, 105, 110, 111–112, 114, 115, 116
American Academy of Family Practice (AAFP)
   on continuity of care, 13, 18
   on immunization schedule, 69
American Academy of Pediatrics (AAP)
   Advisory Committee on Immunization Practices (ACIP), 69, 78
   age-specific preventive-care guidelines recommended by, 85
   on assessing blood pressure in children, 46, 47
   Bright Futures Handbook, 46, 53, 67
   Committee on Infectious Diseases, 43, 69
   establishment of, 4
   investigation to assess clinical effectiveness of number/content of EPSDT/well-child visits, 55
   on managing childhood overweight, 49

medical home definition, 13–14
on number/content of well-child visits, 2, 20, 21, 24, 36, 53, 54, 55, 56, 59, 64, 65, 85, 98, 99, 111, 112, 114, 115
as part of governmental recognition of need for well-child care, 1
recommendation for administration of autism-specific screening tool, 36
recommendation for availability/access to comprehensive preventive care services, 12
recommendation for universal screening for IDA, 41
recommendation for vision screening, 31
recommendation of promotion of continuity of care for patients in all settings, 18
recommendations and utilization of as driven for many years by parental/provider positive expectations rather than empiric evidence of effectiveness, 110
as requesting investigation on clinical effectiveness for well-child care, xi
on SCHIP legislation, 10
screening algorithm of, 33
on tuberculin skin testing (TST), 44
on well-child and preventive-care visits, 53
American Medical Association (AMA), 4
American Thoracic Society, 44
anticipatory guidance, as component of well-child visit. *See* parental anticipatory guidance
asthma, 2, 48, 49, 50, 62, 96, 111
attention-deficit/hyperactivity disorder (ADHD), 58, 86
auditory brainstem response (ABR), 28
Autism and Developmental Disabilities Monitoring (ADDM) (CDC), 36
autism screening, 35–37
autism spectrum disorders (ASDs), 35, 36–37

B

Balanced Budget Act of 1997 (BBA of '97), 10, 11, 85, 89, 90, 102
behavioral problems, 19, 33, 58, 86
Bice, T. W., 21
biotinidase deficiency, 26*t*
block grant funding, 8–9, 10
blood lead levels (BLLs), 37–38, 39, 40
blood pressure (BP), 45
blood pressure screening, 45–48

Blue Cross/Blue Shield, 103
body mass index (BMI), 48, 94
body mass index screening, 48–50
Boxerman, S. B., 21
Boylston, Zebdiel, 68
Bright Futures Handbook (AAP), 46, 53, 67
Bureau of the Census, 71

C

CAD (coronary artery disease), 48
CAH (congenital adrenal hyperplasia), 24, 25t, 27
cardiovascular disease (CVD), 50
care
    continuity of. See continuity of care
    quality of. See quality of care
    without continuity, manifestations of, 19–20
Centers for Disease Control and Prevention (CDC)
    Autism and Developmental Disabilities Monitoring (ADDM), 36
    on BLLs, 37, 38, 39, 40
    growth charts, 49
    on iron deficiency anemia (IDA), 41
    on prevalence of pediatric obesity, 50
    request to Bureau of Census to add questions on poliomyelitis vaccination, 71
    on tuberculin skin testing (TST), 44
Centers for Medicare and Medicaid Services (CMS), 86, 100
central hearing loss, 27, 28
CH (congenital hypothyroidism), 24, 25t, 27
chelation, 40
chest radiograph, 43
child health insurance, 10. See also Medicaid; State Children's Health Insurance Program (SCHIP)
child health, public responsibility for, 4
childhood mortality, effect of well-child care on, 108–109
childhood obesity, 48, 50, 85
Children's Bureau, 1, 3, 5, 11, 12
Children's Defense Fund, 6
CHL (congenital hearing loss), 28, 29
Christakis, D. A., 13
chronic otitis media, 28
citrullinemia type I, 26t
clinical effectiveness
    absence of as not to be construed as evidence of ineffectiveness, 99
    difficulty in confirmation of, 107–110
    early studies of, 106–107
    lack of objective evidence confirming, 66, 99
    need for continued investigation into, 97
    of parental anticipatory guidance, 57, 58, 60, 61–62, 65, 99, 115

paucity of empirical data documenting, 87
recent findings of, 110–111
of routine immunizations birth to six years, 75–78
of well-child care, 55–59
Clinton, Bill, 9
Clinton Health Security Plan, 7
CMS (Centers for Medicare and Medicaid Services), 86, 100
combination vaccines, 19, 69, 70
Committee on Infectious Diseases (AAP), 43, 69
community resources, use of, as opportunity to improve well-child care, 97
compulsory vaccination, 68–69
conductive hearing loss, 27, 29
congenital adrenal hyperplasia (CAH), 24, 25t, 27
congenital hearing loss (CHL), 28, 29
congenital hypothyroidism (CH), 24, 25t, 27
congenital rubella syndrome vaccine, 76t, 79t
connectivity, increase of as opportunity improve well-child care, 95
continuity of care
defined, 13
as enhancing quality, 17–19
studies about, 20–21
coronary artery disease (CAD), 48
cost-effectiveness, of well-child care, 110–111, 113–115
Current Population Survey, 71
CVD (cardiovascular disease), 50

D

Darden, Paul M., 116
Deficit Reduction Act (DRA)
of 1996, 10
of 2005, 90
Department of Health and Human Services (DHHS), 100
depression, 15, 48, 58, 86
developmental and social functioning, effect of well-child care on, 109
developmental delay, 26t, 27, 33, 34–35
developmental screening, 2, 33–35, 36, 87, 97
developmental surveillance, 33, 34
diabetes mellitus (DM), 45, 50
diphtheria, tetanus, and pertussis (DTP) vaccine, 69, 70, 79t
diphtheria vaccine, 70, 74, 76t
down syndrome, 36
DTaP vaccine, 70, 72, 73, 75, 77
DTP/DT/DTaP, 72, 74t
dyslipidemia, 45, 48

E

early and periodic screening, diagnosis, and treatment (EPSDT)
AAP recommendation for, 2
components of, 98
content of, 53
elements of, 88
establishment of, 88, 101

first congressional confrontation regarding, 7–9
impact of Medicaid service delivery changes on, 90
as Medicaid well-child benefit, 1, 5–6, 11, 53, 98
purpose of, 88
and SCHIPs, 10–11
underuse of by Medicaid-enrolled preschool children, 55, 99
electronic medical records, as opportunity to improve well-child care, 95
elevated BLL (EBLL), 39
emergency department (ED) services/visits, 3, 20, 21, 56, 60, 62, 63, 65, 86–87, 93, 105, 108, 110, 111–113, 114, 115, 116
encephalopathy, 40
endocrine diseases (of newborns), 24
evidence-based medicine, parental anticipatory guidance and, 59–65
Expert Panel on Integrated Guidelines for Cardiovascular Health and Risk Reduction in Children and Adolescents, 46
extraimmunization, 19, 20
eye examinations, 30, 32. *See also* vision screening

F

Families USA, 8
Federal Drug Administration (FDA), 55, 107
federal financial participation (FFP), 100
fee-for-service (FFS) model, 61, 100, 103, 106, 110, 111, 113–114
"Fiscal and Healthcare Challenges" (GAO) (2007), 86–87
Fragile X, 36

G

galactosemia, 24, 25*t*
G-codes (Medicare services), 86, 87, 95
government
recognition of need for well-child care by, 1
role of in well-child care, 87–91
-sponsored health care, uneasiness and opposition to, 4
Government Accountability Office (GAO), 86

H

Haemophilus influenzae type b (Hib) vaccine, 69, 72, 73, 74*t*, 75, 76*t*, 79*t*
Health Care Financing Administration (HCFA), 100
Health Information Exchange, 95

health maintenance organizations (HMOs), 103, 111, 113, 114
health-care delivery, impact of increased Medicaid eligibility on, 91
health-care providers, on lack of confirmed clinical effectiveness of well-child care, 57
health-service use, parental anticipatory guidance and long-term health-service use, 62–63
HealthyPeople 2020, 71, 72, 73
hearing, screening for, 27–30
hearing loss, 27–29
hemoglobin (Hgb) levels, 41
hemoglobin SS disease, 24, 25
hepatic steatosis, 48
Hepatitis A (HepA) vaccine, 70, 73, 74t, 75, 76t, 79t
Hepatitis B (HepB) vaccine, 69, 72, 73, 74t, 75, 76t, 79t
Hgb SC disease, 24
Hib (*Haemophilus influenzae* type b) vaccine, 69, 72, 73, 74t, 75, 76t, 79t
HMOs (health maintenance organizations), 103, 111, 113, 114
homocystinuria, 24, 26t
hospitalists, 92, 93
hospitalization, effect of well-child care on, 109
House Select Committee on Children, 6
human immunodeficiency viral infection (HIV), 58
hypercholesterolemia, 48
hyperinsulinemia, 49
hypertension (HTN), 15, 45, 46, 47, 48, 49, 50, 51
hypertriglyceridemia, 49

I

ID (iron deficiency) screening, 41–42
IDA (iron deficiency anemia), 41, 42
immunization registries, 19
immunizations
    clinical effectiveness of, 75–78
    as component of well-child visit, 53, 55, 98
    delivery of, 70–71
    economic impact of, 78–79
    effectiveness of, 107
    goals for delivery of, 71–75
    history of, 68–69
    schedule of, 69–70
    schedule of (1983), 80f
    schedule of (1995), 81f
    schedule of (2006), 81f
    schedule of (2013), 82f
    types of vaccines, 69–70. *See also specific* vaccines
inactivated polio vaccine (IPV), 69, 70
income inequality, in US, 96
influenza vaccine, 70
injury prevention topics, 54
Institute of Medicine (IOM)
    findings on correction of underuse of needed health-care services, 57

quality of care definition, 13, 14–16, 115
reports, xi, 113
insulin resistance, 48, 49, 50
insurance administrators, on lack of confirmed clinical effectiveness of well-child care, 57
intussusception, 70
IPV (inactivated polio vaccine), 69, 70
iron deficiency anemia (IDA), 41, 42
iron deficiency (ID) screening, 41–42

J

Jacobson vs. Commonwealth of Massachusetts, 68

K

Kaiser Permanente, 103

L

language, early intervention strategies for, 35
LaRosa, A. C., 34
latent tuberculosis, 43, 45
lead poisoning screening, 37–41
left ventricular hypertrophy, 48
low HDL cholesterol, 49
low-income children
governmental funding for well-child care for, 1
inadequate preventive care, poor health, and lack of school readiness as disproportionately shared by, 52
lack of medical home by, 3
Medicaid EPSDT/well-child benefits as underutilized by, 2, 99, 101
physical, mental, and developmental preventive-care needs of, 88

M

M. africanum, 43
M. bovis, 43
M. tuberculosis, 43
M. tuberculosis complex, 43
managed care
defined, 103–104
strengths and weaknesses of, 106
managed-care model, 100, 104, 106, 111
Mantoux method, 44
maple syrup urine disease (MSUD), 24, 27t
Marks, K. P., 34
maternal and child health (MCH) activities, 4
maternal-infant bonding, assessment of, 93
Maternity and Infancy Act, 4
Mather, Cotton, 68

MCAD deficiency (medium-chain acyl-CoA dehydrogenase deficiency), 24, 26t
M-CHAT, 36, 37
measles, cases of, 75, 77, 80
measles, mumps, and rubella (MMR) vaccine, 69, 72, 73, 74t, 75, 79t
measles vaccine, 76t, 77, 84f
Medicaid
    child-care focus of in 1965, 88
    as component of public health insurance for children, 12
    eligibility for, 89–90, 101–102
    EPSDT/well-child benefit of, 2. See also early and periodic screening, diagnosis, and treatment (EPSDT)
    establishment of, 100
    expansion of eligibility for, 89, 97
    health-care costs for children enrolled in as greater in preschool years than for privately insured children of same age, 105
    history of, 100–105
    impact of increased eligibility on health-care delivery, 91–95
    managed care to control cost, 102–105
    as part of governmental recognition of need for well-child care, 1
    preschool children insured by as underusing EPSDT and well-child visits, 54
    primary goal of, 100
    reform of, 8–10
    role of, 5–7
    role of in well-child care, 87–91
    states' managerial control with, 91
    strengths and weaknesses of managed care, 106
medical home
    benefits of, 13, 116
    defined, 13–14
    as enhancing quality, 17–19
    lack of, 3, 110
    primary care patient-centered medical homes (PCMH), 92, 118
Medical Home Programs, 91
Medicare
    as entirely federally funded, 91
    as guaranteeing coverage of all eligible individuals, 8
    role of in transforming health-care delivery system, 86
medium-chain acyl-CoA dehydrogenase deficiency (MCAD deficiency), 24, 26t
metabolic disorders (of newborns), 24
metabolic syndrome, 45, 48, 49
MMR (measles, mumps, and rubella) vaccine, 69, 72, 73, 74t, 75, 79t
MSUD (maple syrup urine disease), 24, 27t

multicultural society, impact of on well-child care, 58–59

N

National Academy of Sciences, 14
National Association of Children's Hospitals, 8
National Committee on Infant Mortality, 6
National Governors Association (NGA), 7, 8, 9, 10
National Health and Nutrition Examination Survey (NHANES), 38, 39, 42, 49
National Health Interview Survey (NHIS), 71, 73
National Heart, Lung, and Blood Institute (NHLBI), 46, 47
National High Blood Pressure Education Program Working Group on High Blood Pressure in Children and Adolescents, 45
National Immunization Survey (NIS), 71, 73, 74
newborn screening
for hearing loss, 27–30
for metabolic and other conditions, 23–27
for vision conditions, 30

O

OAE (otoacoustic emission) testing, 28
obesity, 45, 48, 49, 58, 85, 86, 94. *See also* childhood obesity
obstructive sleep apnea, 48
Omnibus Budget Reconciliation Act
of 1981 (OBRA '81), 103
of 1989 (OBRA '89), 7, 11
oral polio vaccine (OPV), 69, 70
otitis media, 28, 76
otitis media with effusion, 29
otoacoustic emission (OAE) testing, 28
overvaccination, 19
overweight, 48, 49

P

paralytic polio, 75
parental anticipatory guidance
clinical effectiveness of, 57, 58, 60, 61–62, 65, 99, 115
as component of well-child visit, 1, 2, 20, 52, 53–54, 55, 56, 58, 60, 92, 98
discrepant thinking regarding clinical effectiveness of, 58–59
and evidence-based medicine, 59–65
and long-term health-service use, 62–63
perspective of health-care providers regarding, 57
perspective of parents and their children regarding, 58
perspective of public- and private-insurance administrators regarding, 57
purpose of, 108

and school readiness, 63–65
parental health education, as
    component of well-child visit,
    56, 57, 66, 108, 111
parental safety measures, 54
parenting skills, assessment of, 93
Partnership for Prevention, 78
patient-centered medical homes
    (PCMH), 92, 118
PCCM (primary care case
    management) plan, 111
PCPs (primary care physicians)
    concern about adequate
        supply of in future, 91
    increasing number of
        as employed by
        hospitals, 92
    initial infant well-child visit, 93
    referred to as private-sector
        physicians, 92
    use of "made sense" or
        "should work effectively"
        approaches, 59
    well-child care training for, 85
PCV (pneumococcal conjugate)
    vaccine, 70, 72, 73, 74t, 75,
    76t, 79t
pediatric obesity, 49–50
Pediatric Tuberculosis
    Collaborative Group, 43
Personal Responsibility and Work
    Opportunity Reconciliation
    Act (PRWORA) (1996),
    89, 90
pertussis
    cases of, 77
    current level of, 75
    incidence of (1980–2010), 84f

phenylketonuria (PKU), 24, 26t, 27
physician and office staff
    education, as opportunity to
    improve well-child care, 97
Plotkin, Stanley, 67
Plotkin, Susan, 67
pneumococcal conjugate (PCV)
    vaccine, 70, 72, 73, 74t, 75,
    76t, 79t
policy, and opportunities to
    improve well-child care,
    95–97
polio vaccine, 69, 71, 72, 73, 74t,
    76t, 79t
poliovirus vaccine, 72, 73, 74t, 75
poverty, US children living in, 96
PPD (purified protein
    derivative), 44
prehypertension, 45, 47
preventive care, ambivalence
    regarding, 58
Preventive Pediatrics (Veeder), 5
preventive-care benefits/programs,
    5, 6, 11, 65, 89
preventive-care visits, 53, 56,
    62, 112
primary care case management
    (PCCM) plan, 111
primary care physicians (PCPs)
    concern about adequate
        supply of in future, 91
    increasing number of
        as employed by
        hospitals, 92
    initial infant well-child visit, 93
    referred to as private-sector
        physicians, 92

use of "made sense" or "should work effectively" approaches, 59
well-child care training for, 85
private sector, role of in well-child care, 92–95
private-insurance policies, as rarely offering coverage for well-child care or requiring co-payment, 99
privately insured children
   percent receiving recommended number of EPSDT and well-child visits in first three years of life, 65
   as underusing EPSDT and well-child visits, 54
   as underusing well-child care, 2
PRWORA (Personal Responsibility and Work Opportunity Reconciliation Act) (1996), 89, 90
pseudostrabismus, 30
ptosis, 30
Public Health Service, 71
purified protein derivative (PPD), 44

Q

quality care, defined, 115–116
quality of care
   defined, 14–17
   studies about, 20–21

R

Radecki, L., 33
referrals, as opportunity to improve well-child care, 95
refractive error, 31
reimbursement incentives, alignment of, as opportunity to improve well-child care, 97
Rodewald, L. E., 78
Roosevelt, Theodore, 3
Rotavirus vaccine, 70, 73, 74t, 75, 76t, 77, 79t
rubella, 75

S

safety measures, for parents, 54
scarlet fever vaccine, 70
SCHIP (State Children's Health Insurance Program), 1, 10–11, 12, 89, 90, 102
school readiness
   impact of receipt of AAP-recommended well-child visits on, 21, 61, 66
   impact of underuse of EPSDT on, 55
   lack of as public health concern, 112
   lack of in low-income children, 52
   lack of in Medicaid-insured children, 110
   parental anticipatory guidance and, 63–65

screening
- autism screening, 35–37
- benefits of, 27
- blood pressure screening, 45–48
- body mass index screening, 48–50
- of children three years and older, 31
- as component of well-child visit, 53, 55, 57, 98
- developmental screening, 33–35
- hearing screening, 27–30
- of infants/toddlers, 31
- iron deficiency (ID) screening, 41–42
- lead poisoning screening, 37–41
- of newborns, 23–30
- tuberculin skin testing (TST), 43–45
- vision screening, 30–32

sensorineural hearing loss, 27–28
service redundancy, decrease of, as opportunity to improve well-child care, 97
Sheppard-Towner Act, 1, 3–5, 11
Sheppard-Towner clinics, 4
sickle cell anemia, 24, 25t, 61
sleep apnea, 48, 50
smallpox, 67, 68, 75
smallpox vaccine, 67, 68, 69, 70–71, 76t
speech, early intervention strategies for, 35
stakeholders, discrepant thinking regarding clinical effectiveness of parental anticipatory guidance, 58
State Children's Health Insurance Program (SCHIP), 1, 10–11, 12, 89, 90, 102
strabismus, 30, 31, 32
Supplemental Security Income (SSI) program, 89

T

Taft, William Howard, 3
Tdap vaccine, 77
Temporary Assistance for Needy Families (TANF) program, 90
tuberculin skin testing (TST), 43–45
tuberculosis (TB), 43
tuberous sclerosis, 36, 46
typhoid fever vaccine, 70
tyrosinemia, 26t

U

United States
- child mortality in compared to other developed countries, 96
- children living in poverty and exposed to income inequality, 96
- as currently at historic vaccination levels, 73
- economic impact of immunization, 78, 79t
- effect of introduction of measles vaccine, 84f
- elimination of rubella, 75

eradication of smallpox, 69
first immunization law, 68
as having second-most expensive health-care system in world, 96
health-care measures, 96
immunization schedule, 70, 80f, 81f, 82f
impact of vaccines, 76t
licensing of measles vaccine, 77
longevity ranking, 96
percent of children categorized as obese, 50
percent of children eligible for Medicaid, 91
percent of children enrolled in Medicaid (prior to 2013), 90
percent of children with developmental delay, 34
percent of children with hypertension, 46
pertussis incidence by year, 84f
prevalence of iron deficiency and IDA, 42
prevalence of lead poisoning, 39
tuberculosis cases, 44
vaccination coverage levels among children 19–35 months (2011), 74t
vaccination coverage levels of preschool children (1967 through June 2011), 83f
well-child care in changing US delivery system, 85–97

universal care policy for children, consideration of, as opportunity to improve well-child care, 96
US Health in International Perspective, 96
US Immunization Survey (USIS), 71, 73
US Morbidity Study, 70
US Preventive Services Task Force (USPSTF), 29, 32, 47, 78, 86

V

vaccine series complete, 72
vaccines. *See also* immunizations
    impact of in the United States, 76t
    types of, 69–70
varicella vaccine, 70, 72, 73, 74t, 75, 76t, 79t
Veeder, Borden, 5
vision screening, 31–32

W

Walker, David, 86
well-child care
    anticipatory guidance component of. *See* parental anticipatory guidance
    assessing effectiveness of, 55–56. *See also* clinical effectiveness
    association of with health-service utilization, 61

barrier to provision and
utilization of, 87
benefits of, 2–3
components of, 1–3
future needs for, 11–12
government role in, 87–91
history of, 3–11
Medicaid-insured children as
underusing, 54
policy and opportunities to
improve on, 95–97
prioritizing recommended
topics for, 92–95
private sector role in, 92–95
privately insured children as
underusing, 2
as prudent investment for
future, 116
quasi-standardization of,
87–88
studies about, 20–21
unproven benefits of as
clear, 60
utilization of, 57–59
well-child clinics, establishment
of, 5

well-child visits
AAP-recommended number/
content of. See
American Academy of
Pediatrics (AAP)
benefits of, 2
components/content of, 1, 33,
36, 44, 53
description, 53–56
initial infant well-child visit,
24, 93
White House Conference on
Children, 3
whooping cough, 77
World Health Organization, 116

Y

Youth and Families, 6

Z

Zhou, C., 78

Made in the USA
Columbia, SC
29 January 2021